FAST-FIX
GI
DIET

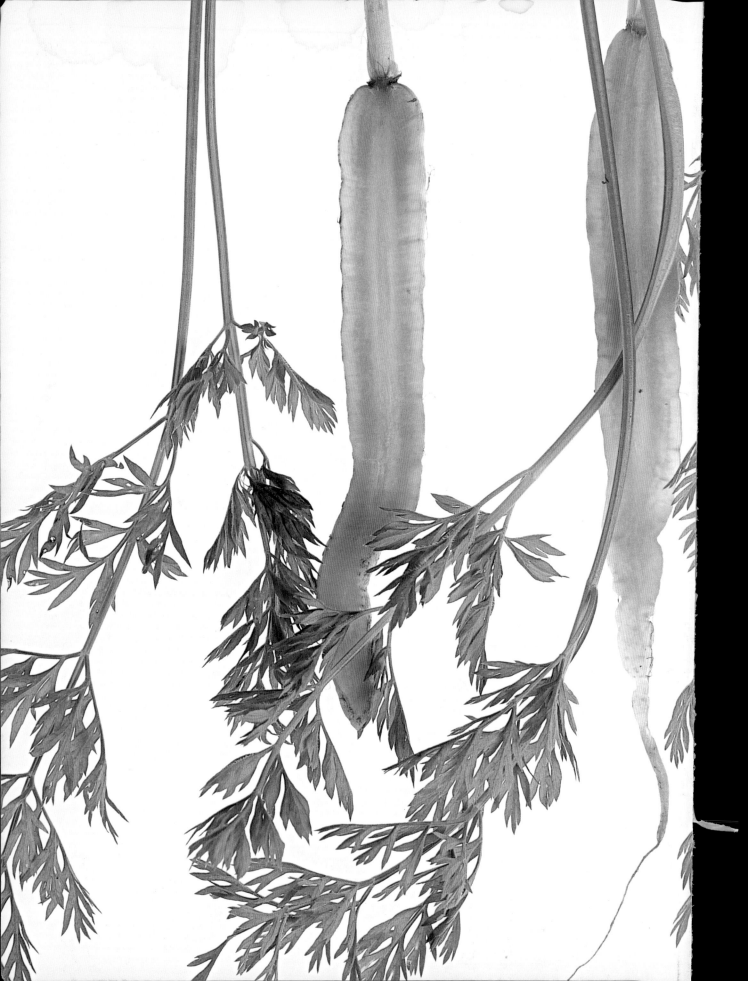

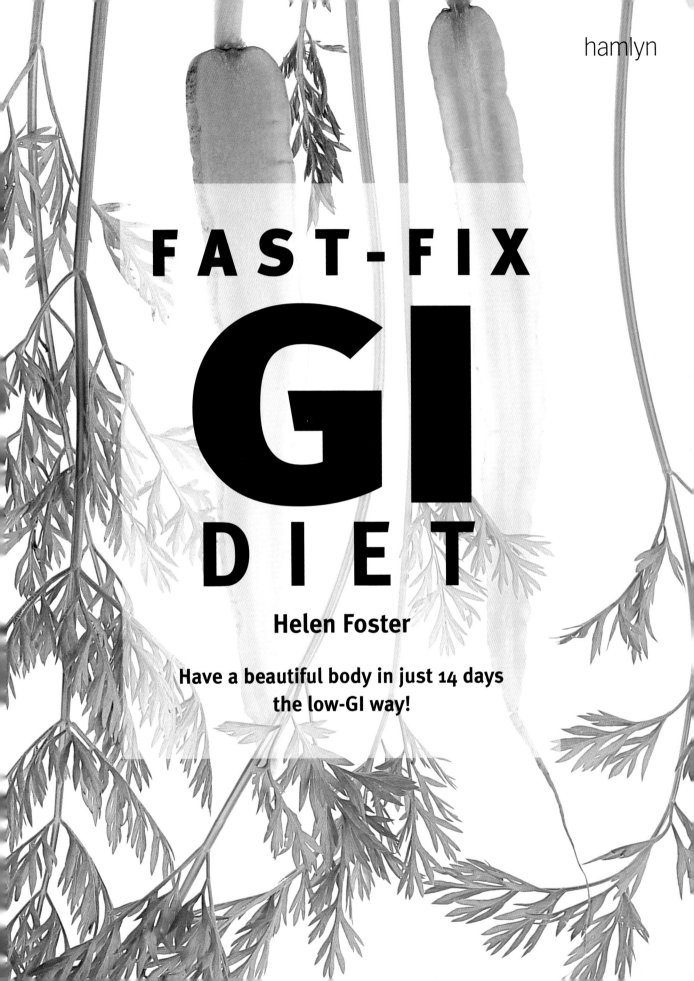

hamlyn

FAST-FIX
GI
DIET

Helen Foster

**Have a beautiful body in just 14 days
the low-GI way!**

Notes

It is advisable to check with your doc[tor]
or diet plan. The advice given in this [book is no]
replacement for professional medical treatment. While the information
given here is believed to be accurate and the step-by-step instructions
have been devised to avoid strain, neither the author nor the publisher can
accept any legal responsibility to any injury or illness sustained while
following the exercises and diet plan.

Ovens should be preheated to the specified temperature. If using a fan-
assisted oven, follow the manufacturer's instructions for adjusting the time
and temperature. Broilers should also be preheated.

This book includes dishes made with nuts and nut derivatives. It is
advisable for those with known allergic reactions to nuts and nut
derivatives and those who may be potentially vulnerable to these allergies,
such as pregnant and nursing mothers, invalids, the elderly, babies and
children, to avoid dishes made with nuts and nut oils. It is also prudent to
check the labels of preprepared ingredients for the possible inclusion of
nut derivatives.

Meat and poultry should be cooked thoroughly. To test if poultry is cooked,
pierce the flesh through the thickest part with a skewer or fork—the juices
should run clear, never pink or red.

All the recipes in this book have been analyzed by a professional nutritionist.
The analysis refers to each portion without serving suggestions.

First published in Great Britain in 2006 by
Hamlyn, a division of Octopus Publishing Group Ltd
2–4 Heron Quays, London E14 4JP

Copyright © Octopus Publishing Group Ltd 2006

Distributed in the United States and Canada by
Sterling Publishing Co., Inc.
387 Park Avenue South, New York, NY 10016--8810

ISBN-13: 978-0-600-61500-2
ISBN-10: 0-600-61500-6

A CIP catalogue record for this book is available from
the British Library.

Printed and bound in China

10 9 8 7 6 5 4 3 2 1

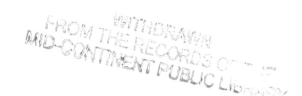

contents

Introduction

one of the most frustrating things about weight loss is that generally you have to make a choice.

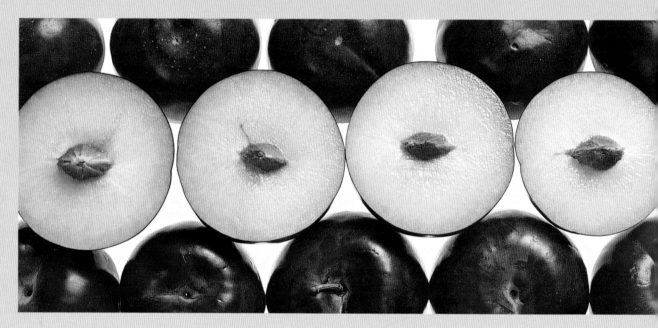

Do you follow one of the faddy diets that cut out entire food groups and come with some worrying side-effects but trigger weight loss quickly enough that every time you step on the scales you smile? Or do you go the sensible route, choosing a healthy eating plan where no food is banned, but weight loss is slow and steady? The latter option is great for long-term results, but not so helpful if you're going on vacation in two weeks' time, have a special occasion to go to (and a special outfit to get into), or simply want a motivating burst to kick-start your way onto a longer term weight-loss program. Picking up this book is the first step toward ending that frustration because you won't have to make those choices. For the first time you can eat a healthy, sensible diet with no faddy foods, no starvation, and plenty of healthy fruit, vegetables, and whole grains, and still get results that make you smile when you stand on the scales.

The reason this diet works is that you follow a low-calorie eating plan based on the sound scientific principles of the Glycemic Index (GI) to trigger steady, safe, sustainable fat loss from your body. In addition, you incorporate some simple toning and cardiovascular exercise to increase that fat loss through aerobic calorie-burning. But things don't end there—this plan also uses daily power-ups that help promote extra weight loss by fighting problems such as a sluggish metabolism, excess fluid, and poor posture, which can undermine your weight-loss efforts. The result is that in the 14 days on which you follow this diet you can shed up to 6½ pounds—and lose inches from your hips, tummy, and thighs.

However, there are more benefits to this diet than weight loss alone. The Glycemic Index is one of the most exciting areas of nutritional science today. All over the world researchers are investigating the positive health benefits of this simple eating approach and are concluding that eating primarily foods with a low GI can positively influence the health and well-being of every cell in your body. By balancing levels of vital blood sugars, fats, and hormones through eating the low-GI way, you create the ideal biological conditions in your body for higher energy levels, positive emotional sensations, and all-round general health and longevity.

It's no surprise, therefore, that so many people who start on a low-GI plan (even a short one like this) want to follow its principles for life. And that's where the final benefit of this fast-fix plan reveals itself. While many diet plans—particularly those of the rapid-results variety—leave you high and dry when the plan is over, on this diet you'll learn everything you need to help you continue to follow this healthy way for life.

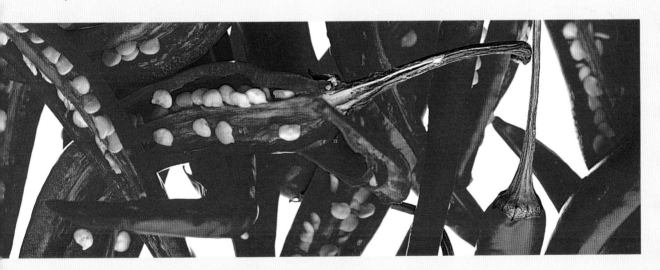

The result? The next 14 days could be the most important of your life so far for your health.

What is GI?

GI is possibly the most important term you need to know about if you want to lose weight today. It stands for Glycemic Index and, put very simply, it's a measure of how fast a food turns to the sugar known as glucose (which you use as fuel) in your body. A food that converts quickly is known as a high-GI food, while one that converts slowly is known as a low-GI food.

Admittedly, it's not a new concept—the Glycemic Index (GI) has been known about for more than two decades (primarily as a way to help diabetics control their insulin levels)—but only recently has the role of GI in weight loss been explored extensively enough to determine its importance.

In the last few years, studies have discovered that:

1 Switching from high-GI foods to low-GI alternatives actually revs up your metabolic rate, increasing the number of calories that you burn each day by 4 percent, and this alone could see the average woman losing around 8 pounds a year and the average man losing around 10½ pounds a year with no further alterations to their diet. But, more importantly for dieters, this metabolic boost dramatically reduces the normal slowdown that occurs when you cut your calorie intake.

2 Low-GI foods also boost fat-burning. According to a study published in the journal *Nutrition and Metabolism*, the presence of the low-GI form of starch (known

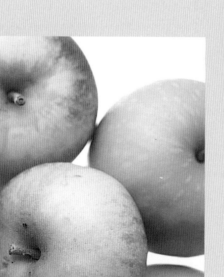

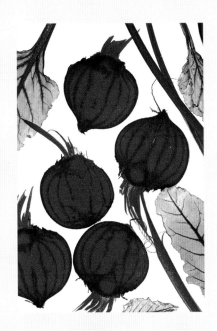

as amylose) in your diet actually triggers fat-burning after eating—and it can, in high enough quantities, rev up the speed at which you do this by 23 percent. Eating a low-GI meal before exercise has also been shown to increase the amount of fat that you burn during your workout.

3 People who switch even just the white bread in their diet to a lower GI alternative gain roughly one-third fewer inches around their waist every single year than those who eat higher GI white breads, says US-based GI researcher Dr Katherine Tucker in the *American Journal of Clinical Nutrition*. One reason for this could be that the low-GI eaters produce less insulin (which just loves to store excess calories around the abdomen)

than the white-bread eaters. And it's believed that switching to an overall low-GI diet could have an even greater effect.

4 When you switch to eating the low-GI way, your appetite naturally decreases, making weight loss easier than it's ever been before. In a trial proving the metabolic boost of GI eating, researchers also discovered that the dieters felt considerably less hungry than those who were not eating the low-GI way. This echoes past research, which found that the appetite was naturally kept in check on a low-GI diet—in fact, after eating a low-GI meal, volunteers in a trial at Tufts University in Boston, US, consumed 81 percent fewer calories at their next meal without noticing, thereby dramatically boosting their weight-loss efforts.

5 Eating low-GI foods makes exercise feel easier. Exercise is a vital part of weight loss, and eating the low-GI way actually aids exercise. In a trial undertaken by Case Western University in Ohio, US, women given a low-GI meal before they worked out managed to last 16 percent longer in exercise tests than high-GI eaters, because they had much more energy with which to sustain their efforts.

Because of these factors many nutritionists now believe that eating the low-GI way is the healthiest—and, potentially, the most effective—way to lose weight and to keep it off for life. But to understand how to do this properly, you need to know exactly how food acts in your body and what makes a food high-GI or low-GI.

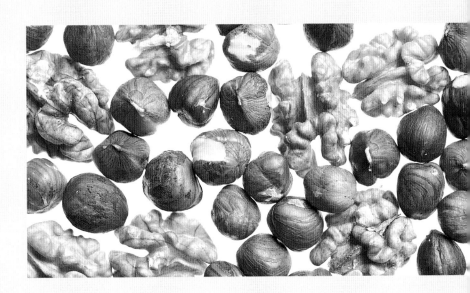

GI explained

When you eat a food that contains carbohydrate, that food is converted by your body into a sugar called glucose, which your body uses as energy. The faster a food makes this conversion, the faster sugar enters your system. If you're an athlete who suddenly needs to replenish his or her sugar stores, this is a good thing; however, if you're a sedentary office worker, a sudden rise in glucose levels might not be so positive.

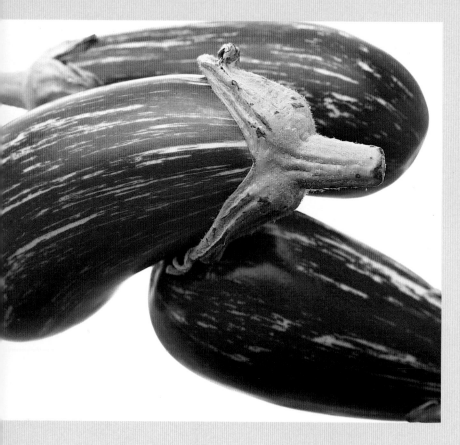

The reason is that if too much glucose is released into your system in one go, your body panics. The result is a rapid release of another hormone, known as insulin, which then shuttles the extra sugar out of your system and into the fat stores. This alone contributes to weight gain—particularly around the abdominal area, where, as mentioned on page 9, insulin has a particular fondness for depositing extra sugar. But to compound the problem, this initial reaction triggers a knock-on nutritional effect.

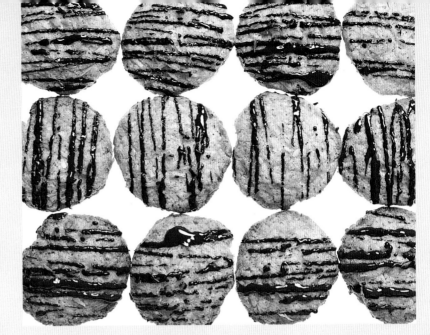

You see, after insulin has done its job, blood-sugar levels in the body are left low—often too low to provide your organs, muscles, and brain with all the fuel they need to carry out the myriad tasks demanded of them every hour. This lack of fuel then causes a different type of panic, which sees the appetite part of the brain sending out strong psychological signals for foods that can help it replenish its fuel stores quickly: psychological signals that you interpret as cravings for chocolate, candy, or easily digested carbohydrates such as white bread and sugary drinks. The result: you eat more high-GI foods and the fat-making circle begins again.

However, switching to low-GI foods stops this vicious circle in its tracks. Low-GI foods convert far more steadily to sugar, eliminating the body's need for a panic reaction and the subsequent sugar cravings to reverse it. The result is that less glucose ends up in your fat stores—and fewer calories end up being consumed to boost your flagging energy levels. These two effects combine to help keep your weight stable. Add calorie control, a little exercise, and some fluid-fighting to the mix (as you're going to do in the 14-day diet plan on pages 24–85) and you have an all-round recipe for weight loss.

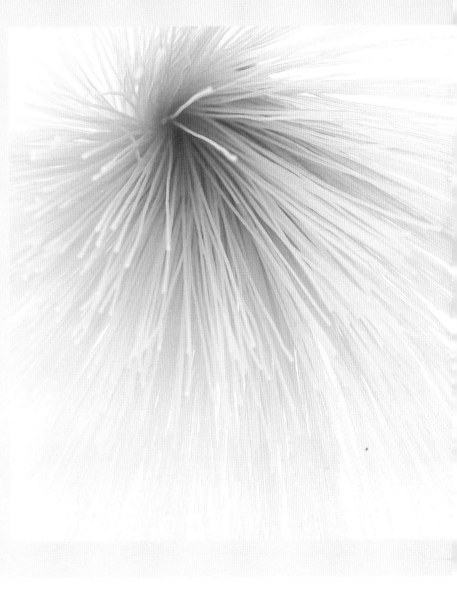

High GI and low GI

Remember, the GI of a food is determined by how fast the amount of carbohydrate in that food converts to sugar within the body. Because of this, foods that don't contain any carbohydrate—such as meat, fish, and poultry (which are pure protein foods) and butter, margarine, and cooking oils (which are pure fat)—are automatically assumed to be low-GI foods.

Having a high level of either protein or fat also dramatically lowers GI, which is why beans, legumes, nuts, seeds, and dairy products that combine high levels of protein or fat with carbohydrates are generally very low-GI foods. However, within carbohydrate foods, GI values can vary widely, and there are two main factors that influence this variation.

the type of sugar that a food contains

A food that contains a high level of glucose (found in manufactured items such as sports drinks and energy candy, and also in naturally sweet fruits like watermelon) will convert very quickly to sugar in the body. Other types of sugar convert more slowly. One reason for this is that many sugars (known as

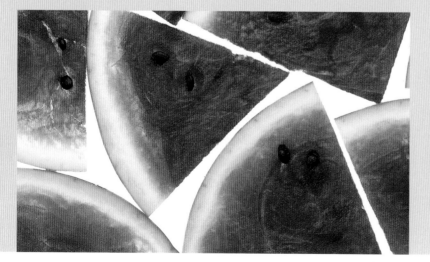

disaccharides) are made up of two molecules (one of glucose, one of fructose), which means they have to be split before they can be effectively converted, thereby considerably slowing the time that the process takes. The disaccharide sugars include sucrose (commonly known as table sugar), lactose (the sugar in dairy products), and maltose (which tends to be used as a flavoring in foods). Fructose (the main sugar in fruit) has only one molecule, but because this has to be changed into glucose before it can be used, it, too, has a low GI.

how easy the food is for your body to break down

Fiber is hard for the body to digest, and so the higher the fiber content of a food, the lower its GI is likely to be. For example, multigrain bread (which contains fragments of wheat still with the husks on) takes far more effort to break down than white bread (from which the fibrous husks have been removed). However, the other elements that affect GI are the type and form of starch it contains. The more resistant to breakdown the starch in a food is, the lower the GI of that food will be. This explains why rice (which doesn't contain much resistant starch) is never a low-GI food, and why pasta (which contains lots of resistant starch) is always low-GI. But it also explains why so many of us eat high-GI diets most of the time. You see, when you process a food, you make the starch particles within it much smaller, making them easier to break down—and allowing faster conversion to glucose. This explains why white bread has a higher GI than whole-wheat bread, and why bran flakes (where the fibrous shell of the bran is crushed while they are shaped) have a higher GI than noodle-shaped bran cereals (which aren't as "squashed").

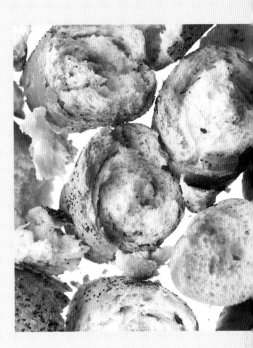

GI at a glance

To measure a food's GI scientists evaluate how fast it converts to sugar compared to glucose. If glucose is 100 on the scale, then any food that converts 70 percent as fast (and above) is said to be a high-GI food; those foods that convert 56–69 percent as fast are medium-GI foods; and those that convert 55 percent (and below) as fast are known as low-GI foods. You'll find the ratings for hundreds of foods in the chart on pages 110–125. Some ratings of common foods include:

High GI foods
- Glucose drinks
- White and whole-wheat bread
- White rice and quick-cook rice
- Mashed potatoes and baked potatoes
- Watermelon
- Parsnips
- Dates

Medium GI foods
- Sucrose (ordinary table sugar, which is used in all sorts of cakes, candies, pastries, and soft drinks)
- Basmati rice and brown rice
- Pineapple
- Beet
- Carrots
- Pita bread
- Pancakes
- Most canned fruits
- Dried figs

Low GI foods
- Oats
- Pasta
- Beans (except fava beans)
- Legumes
- Nuts and seeds
- Grain breads and seeded breads
- Sweet potatoes
- New potatoes
- Apples
- Cherries and berries
- Milk
- Yogurt
- Soy foods, such as tofu, tempeh, and yogurt

The best low-GI foods

One of the reasons many experts believe so strongly in the
health-boosting powers of the GI diet is because it invariably
contains high levels of nutrient-packed fruits, vegetables, and
whole grains. Simply following any low-GI diet will help improve
your health for this reason, but there are some low-GI foods that
deserve inclusion weekly (if not daily) in your diet plans.

1 berries
Blueberries contain the
highest levels of antioxidants
(substances that neutralize
harmful molecules called free
radicals). However, all berries
are important health-boosters—
raspberries and strawberries,
for example, contain vital
cancer-fighting chemicals.

2 beans and legumes
Studies have shown that diets rich
in beans and legumes (which are
high in fibre and protein) play an
active part in lowering cholesterol
and blood pressure and reducing
the incidence of diabetes. Eating
just four servings a week is
believed to cut the risk of heart
disease by 22 percent.

3 cruciferous vegetables
The vegetables in this family
(which include broccoli, cabbage,
sprouts, and cauliflower) all
contain a vital cancer-prevention
agent called sulforaphane. New
research has revealed that
steaming vegetables releases
more of this agent than boiling,
so steam don't boil!

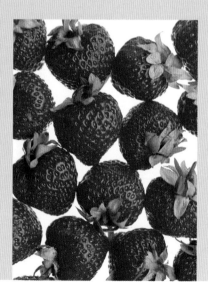
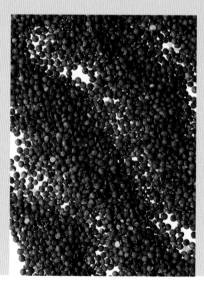
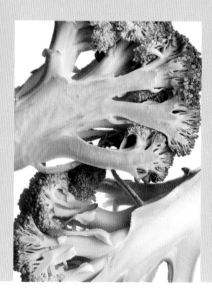

4 dark chocolate

Chocolate is a low-GI food because it contains fat, dairy products, and sucrose—and it's a healthy food because it contains antioxidants. However, only good-quality dark chocolate fits the bill, so look for brands containing 70–80 percent cocoa solids, and stick to just four squares at a time (roughly 100 calories).

6 nuts and seeds

The essential fats in nuts and seeds aren't just linked to a lower risk of heart disease (one handful of nuts per day could cut your risk of heart attack by at least 15 percent). They also create healthy skin, boost your mood, and can even help stimulate fat-burning in the body. They are calorific, though, so watch portion sizes closely.

8 quinoa

Many nutritionists say that this grain (which you use as you would rice or couscous) is one of the most complete foods there is. A relative of spinach, quinoa is incredibly high in protein and complex carbohydrates—plus it's packed with energy-giving B vitamins and iron.

9 soy foods

A great source of vegetarian protein, soy is also high in ingredients known as isoflavones, which act like estrogen in the body. This potentially decreases the risk of breast cancer and menopausal problems in women and may protect against prostate cancer in men. Soy also fights heart disease in both genders.

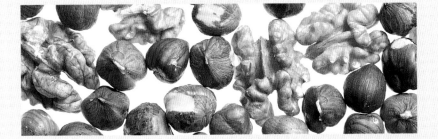

5 herbs and spices

Adding a pinch of rosemary to your food delivers the same antioxidant benefits as eating a handful of berries. And oregano is nine times more potent than rosemary. Spices such as turmeric and cinnamon also have many health benefits, including potentially fighting diabetes.

7 oats

Well known for their ability to lower cholesterol (one bowl of oats a day can cut cholesterol levels by as much as 23 percent), oats also control blood sugar and contain a potent antioxidant called ferulic acid, which is linked to a lower risk of colon cancer.

10 sweet potatoes

Ranked top of all vegetables for their fiber and vitamin content by the US-based Center for Science in the Public Interest, sweet potatoes are packed with vitamins A and C, iron, and copper. You can cook them just as you would normal potatoes: mashed, fried, or roasted.

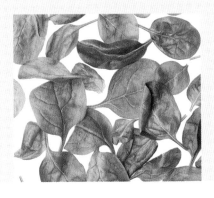

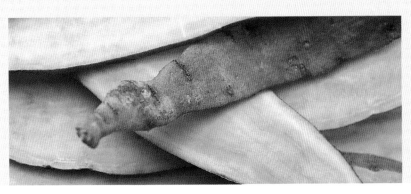

When GI goes bad

Although the list of GI superfoods is beyond reproach, the fact that a high-fat content lowers the GI of a food means that many foods that fit the criteria of healthy in terms of their GI rating have high levels of saturated fat, trans fats, and calories. On top of this, other potentially not-so-healthy foods also come with a very low-GI rating. Foods to watch include:

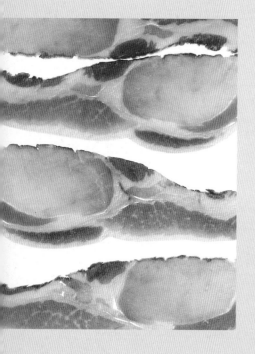

1 bacon, burgers, sausages, etc.

Low-GI because they are packed with protein, these foods do contain high levels of saturated fat, and they are also high in salt, which raises blood pressure and increases the risk of fluid retention. If you want to eat these foods (and other high-fat meats, such as ground meat and duck), remove any obvious fat before cooking, then broil or dry-fry them; before serving, pat the food with paper towel to soak up any surface lipid fats.

2 chips

Low-GI these may be, but low in calories they are not! If you want something to accompany a sandwich or feel like a snack, you'll get a similar crunch sensation (but many, many more nutrients) if you choose crudités like celery or baby carrots—or try a pickle, such as gherkins or pearl onions, which stimulate similar taste receptors to many chip flavors but with a fraction of the calories.

3 coffee

While coffee doesn't technically raise blood sugar, Dutch researchers have determined that it interferes with the way cells respond to insulin, possibly increasing the amount in your system, which in turn increases the risk of fat storage. Decaffeinated coffee doesn't have this effect, so make the switch today. If you feel that you can't do without that caffeine boost first thing in the morning, at least keep your intake of caffeinated blends down to fewer than four cups a day.

4 diet sodas

While no one has proved that artificial sweeteners are bad for you, researchers at Purdue University in Indiana, US, have found that they do confuse your body's satiety systems, making it more likely that you'll overeat. It's ok to drink diet soda once in a while, but better choices are water, green tea, and herbal blends, either drunk hot or cooled and poured over ice.

5 ice cream

Yes, it's delicious, and yes, it contains fat-burning calcium, but ice cream also contains high levels of saturated fat—and the more luxurious the ice cream, the more likely this is. If you want to have an ice-cream dessert once in a while, choose a low-fat variety and serve yourself just one scoop, ideally accompanying it with fruit to boost your nutrient intake and to satiate your appetite.

6 margarine

Many varieties of margarine contain extremely high levels of altered fats known as trans fats, which researchers are now linking to an increased risk of heart disease. Choose varieties that actively say they are trans-fat-free, or use small amounts of butter which may be slightly higher in saturated fat than margarine, but many experts currently believe that this is less harmful than trans fats.

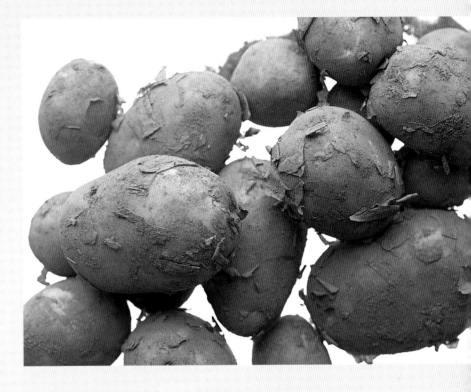

7 spirits

Spirits may be the lowest in GI of any alcoholic drink, but they are also the most potent and are linked to the highest incidence of some digestive cancers and diabetes. Wine may have a slightly higher GI, but if it is drunk as part of a meal or with a small handful of cashews or almonds (which will slow down its sugar conversion), it's a far healthier alcoholic choice.

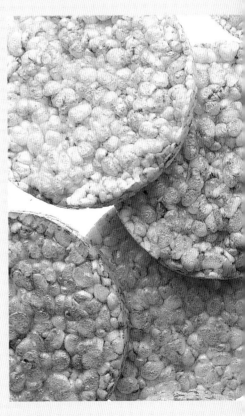

GI health benefits

With so many healthy foods incorporated into eating the low-GI way, it's easy to see that it's going to be good for your health. However, the benefits could be even greater than you believed.

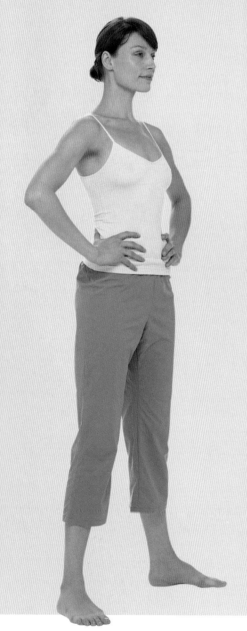

GI fights major illnesses

As we explained on pages 8–9, one of the main problems of a high-GI diet is that it increases the levels of insulin in your body. And this isn't just bad news for your waistline—insulin can be a very harmful substance. Not only is it linked to a higher incidence of diabetes, but high insulin levels also encourage the production of hormones that can promote growth in some cancer cells, with the result that breast and pancreatic cancers have both been linked to high-GI diets. But lowered insulin isn't the only consequence of cutting down on high-GI foods. Studies have also shown that cutting down on refined foods reduces the levels of cholesterol and heart-disease-triggering fats called triglycerides. Finally, researchers in Seoul, South Korea, have discovered that simply swapping one high-GI food for a lower GI equivalent (in this case white rice for other whole grains) reduced levels of the harmful amino acid known as homocysteine. This is incredibly important, because this particular amino acid is known to be linked to heart problems and is believed to be a major contributor to the debilitating condition, Alzheimer's disease.

GI fights minor health problems

By tackling blood-sugar swings, low-GI eating is known to help reduce the effects of pre-menstrual syndrome. It's also linked to a greater control of hormones in general, which could help reduce the risk of a condition called polycystic ovary syndrome as well as other fertility problems. However, a more general benefit is that eating the low-GI way may boost your immune system. When you eat a low-GI diet, the amount of sugar in your body is naturally reduced —which is good news, because sugar is an immune-suppressor. Eating the low-GI way also increases the amount of vitamin C that you are able to absorb from

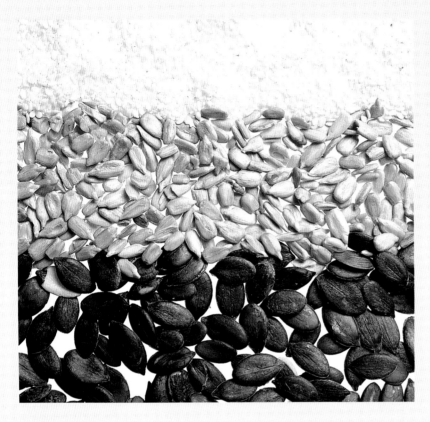

skin. More importantly, high insulin levels in the body have been linked to increased rates of acne and oily skin—and, possibly, to a faster rate of aging. By reducing the levels of insulin in your diet you'll be helping to create healthy skin from within. And because protein foods feature heavily in low-GI diets, your hair will thank you, too. Hair is made from protein, but if you're not getting enough protein in your diet, your hair is the area to which your body will limit supplies. By boosting your protein intake to adequate levels, you could find that in a matter of weeks your hair both looks shinier and feels healthier and thicker.

foods (because vitamin C and glucose compete to enter the body's cells), and it's well known that people with high blood levels of vitamin C are less susceptible to minor ailments such as colds and flu than those with lower levels.

GI boosts your mood and energy

By providing your body with a slow, steady supply of energy, you prevent the peaks and troughs that trigger the mood and energy swings that many people experience throughout the day. In fact, within two or three days of starting to eat the low-GI way you should find that your energy levels improve. In addition to this, you'll also possibly be eating higher levels of carbohydrate foods on this diet plan than you would normally do while slimming, and this is important as it boosts levels in the brain of the mood-enhancing hormone serotonin. Low levels of serotonin have been linked to depression and comfort-eating.

GI enhances your looks

By adding high levels of essential fats (in the form of nuts and seeds) to your diet, you immediately enhance the appearance and health of your

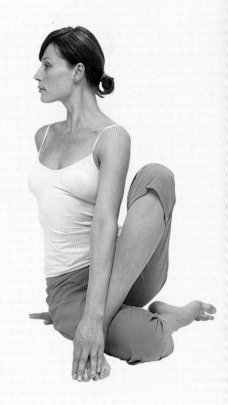

The GI pyramid

Now that you've seen all the positive effects of eating the low-GI way, you're probably wondering what on earth you should be eating (and when) to harness those benefits. Well, the diagram opposite explains everything quickly and simply. It's called the GI pyramid, and it's been designed to show, at a glance, what makes up a healthy low-GI diet.

There are seven layers overall: foods with a high GI (which also contain few additional nutrients) are shown at the top of the pyramid, while foods with a low GI (but high nutrient values) appear at the bottom. Not surprisingly, foods at the top of the pyramid should be severely limited, while several portions of those foods at the bottom should be eaten every day.

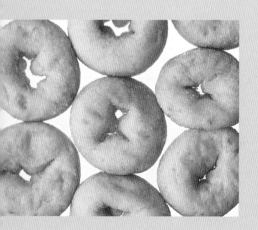

foods at the top of the pyramid

These foods don't just have a high GI; they also contain few additional nutrients or lots of fat. They include glucose drinks, sugary drinks, such as soda, hard candy and similar treats, chips, cakes, cookies, pastries, and sugary puddings. If you eat these at all, make it no more than once a week.

second-layer foods

These include mashed potatoes, white and brown breads, rice, and sugar cereals. They're still very high-GI foods, but they do have some nutrients in them, so they're not totally banned. Restrict servings to one or two a week, though—and always eat them with a low-GI food, which slows down the speed at which they convert to sugar.

third-layer foods

Nuts and seeds have a low GI. They are also a good source of fiber and oils, containing essential fatty acids, so you should aim to have 1 ounce of these each day. You can also include nut- or seed-based products in this category, which means foods like peanut butter and spreads like tahini (made from sesame seeds). Roughly 1½ teaspoons of these products will contain the same number of calories as 1 ounce of nuts or seeds.

fourth-layer foods

These are the pure protein foods, such as red meats (beef, pork, and lamb), poultry (chicken, turkey, duck, and goose), offal (kidneys, heart, and liver), fish (white fish such as cod and flounder, and oily fish such as salmon, herrings, sardines, pilchards, fresh tuna, and trout), shellfish (oysters, crab, shrimp, cockles, and mussels), and eggs. Because they contain no carbohydrates, they have a GI of 0. Aim for two or three portions of these foods a day.

fifth-layer foods

Their combination of protein and the relatively slow-digesting sugar known as lactose make milk and dairy products low-GI foods. They're also an important source of calcium, which isn't just good for your bones—research has proved that it also helps reduce fat storage. Aim for two to three servings of dairy products a day—but choose low-fat varieties to cut down on calories and saturated fat intake.

sixth-layer foods

These foods are the starchy carbohydrates, which should give you your main source of energy. You should eat between six and eleven servings of carbohydrates a day, focusing mainly on low-GI varieties, such as multigrain bread, pasta, oats, grains like barley and quinoa, and sweet or new potatoes. However, if you have already eaten any servings of the starchy carbohydrates (such as white bread and rice) that appear higher up the GI pyramid, then you need to reduce the number of helpings of low-GI foods accordingly.

foods at the bottom of the pyramid

It is recommended that everyone eats at least five portions of fruit and vegetables per day, and virtually all fruit and vegetables have a low GI. There are a few exceptions to this (including watermelon and root vegetables, such as squash or rutabaga), but one of the problems with the GI testing system is that the amount of fruit and vegetables tested is far greater than you would actually eat, meaning that the insulin effect they will actually have in your body is lessened. Because of this, it's now generally agreed that it's ok to eat all fruit and vegetables on a low-GI diet.

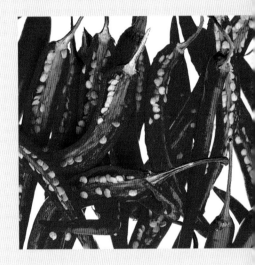

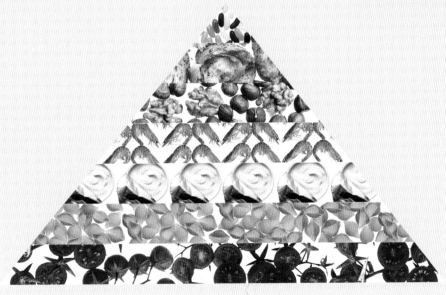

Portion distortion

Although choosing low-GI foods naturally puts your body into a positive state for slimming (remember, your metabolic rate is going to be faster than on any other form of dieting program and you'll be more likely to burn fat by eating the low-GI way), weight loss is always a matter of calories in versus calories out, so portion sizes do count.

The GI pyramid on page 21 indicates the overall proportions of the different food groups that you should eat each day. Now you'll learn how big that portion should actually be, to fit the diet plan that follows.

• **Bread:** 1 slice of a loaf; half a small roll/bagel

• **Breakfast cereal:** 1 oz—roughly 3 tablespoons

• **Butter and spreads**—enough to cover the tip of a knife

• **Cheese:** 1½ oz—a piece the size of a matchbox

• **Eggs:** one medium-sized egg

• **Fish:** 5 oz—the size of a checkbook but slightly thicker

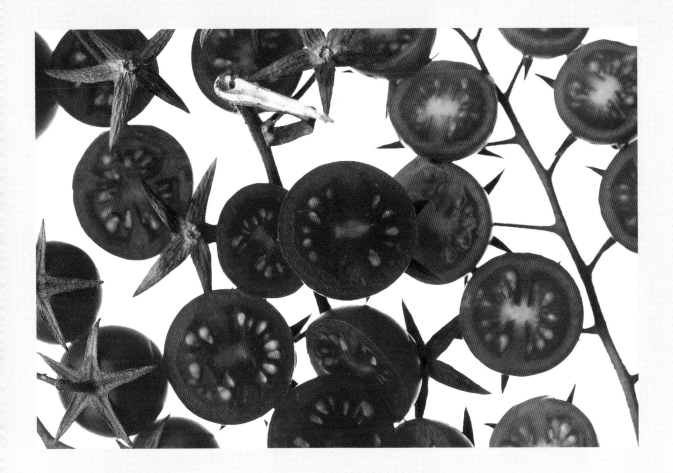

- **Fruit:** one medium piece (such as an apple or orange); two small pieces of fruit, such as kiwi; enough berries to fit in two cupped hands; or one-eighth of a large fruit, such as a watermelon

- **Fruit juice:** ⅔ cup—that's roughly three fingers high in a small glass

- **Meat:** 4 oz—the size of a deck of cards

- **Milk (dairy or soy):** ¾ cup— that's roughly four fingers high in a small glass

- **Nuts and seeds:** 3 tablespoons —enough to fit in the palm of a cupped hand

- **Oils:** ½ tablespoon, but it's better to use an oil spray, which cuts down on the calories

- **Potatoes:** 4 oz—that means an egg-size whole potato, two small boiled potatoes, or roughly 2 heaped tablespoons mashed potato

- **Rice, pasta, couscous:** 2 tablespoons uncooked—that's roughly one large serving spoonful when cooked

- **Shellfish:** 5 oz—roughly two cupped hands full of shrimp, mussels, clams, etc.

- **Vegetables:** enough to fit in two cupped hands

- **Yogurt (dairy or soy) or cottage cheese:** one small carton (normally ½ cup)

FAST

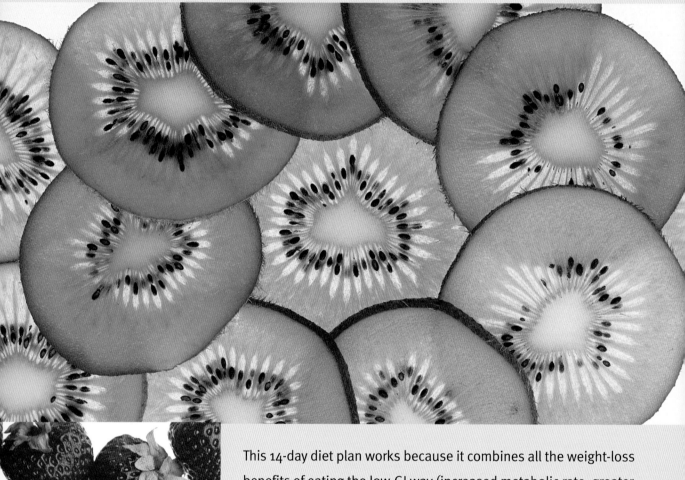

This 14-day diet plan works because it combines all the weight-loss benefits of eating the low-GI way (increased metabolic rate, greater fat metabolism, reduced sugar cravings, and an increase in energy that makes anything seem possible) with simple calorie-burning exercises and power-up tricks. These either make it easier for you to stay motivated or enhance the weight-loss effects of the diet by reducing fluid retention and other problems such as poor posture. After just 14 days on this plan you will notice your changes.

lose weight

The combination of carefully calorie-counted menus, exercise, and increased metabolic stimulation guarantees weight loss of up to 6½ pounds on this program. Together with the feel good tips that you will follow each day, this leads to more rapid weight loss than traditional low-GI plans offer, helping you to achieve your fast-fix aims as easily as possible. As a general rule, the more you weigh to start with, the greater your weight loss will be (because you burn more calories from day to day anyway), but everyone who follows the plan as directed will lose weight.

look and feel thinner

A combination of weight loss, better posture, and light muscle toning will ensure you start to lose inches around the tummy, hips, and thighs. If you really want to track your progress, wrap a piece of string round your waist before the diet starts (either mark with a pen where the two ends meet or snip the string to fit); at the end of the two weeks, try this again—it's almost certain the string will be too big.

improve your skintone

As we have already mentioned on page 19, better skin is a major benefit of eating the low-GI way, and within just two weeks of increasing your daily intake of essential fats, cutting down on sugars, and boosting your intake of fluids, you will plump up dehydrated skin on your face and body, giving you a head-to-toe glow.

reduce signs of cellulite

Cellulite is a combination of fat and fluid, and by helping you lose weight and flush out fluid (together with toning exercises that firm the muscles under those lumps and bumps) this diet could help mild cases of cellulite vanish within two weeks. More serious cases will take longer, but the increased hydration of your skin will definitely make cellulite less noticeable while you concentrate on defeating those stubborn areas for good.

So that's it: a head-to-toe body make-over in just 14 days. Of course, to get results you need to follow the plan as directed, so read on to discover exactly what you need to do and when.

need some extra help?

If you've got more than 6½ pounds to lose (or just love the effects of this fast-fix GI diet so much that you want to keep going when the 14 days are over), that's no problem. You can either repeat the diet exactly as it is or chop and change things, using the alternative options suggested with the recipes. For meals where no alternative is given, remember that you can always swap like for like on a diet—so, any fruit can be replaced by another fruit; any vegetable can be swapped for another vegetable; any meat can be swapped for meat, fish, or poultry in the same-size portion; and you can swap any carbohydrate for another low-GI carb as well.

What to do and when

The 14-day plan that follows includes three main elements: "food," "fit" and "feel good." Each is explained in greater detail below, but every day the minimum you should do is eat the meals and snacks suggested and carry out the toning exercises that appear on pages 90–103. The "fit" and "feel good" tips will help boost your results, so try and incorporate as many of them as possible.

food

Every day you'll find three main meals and two snacks to eat. This may actually be more food than you're used to eating (especially when you're trying to slim), but don't skip any meal or snack. Eating regularly actually boosts weight loss, by fooling your body into thinking it's eating more than it is, so preventing the metabolic slowdown that usually occurs when you cut calories. You'll notice that each day there is a recipe to follow or an easy-to-make alternative if you don't fancy cooking that day. Don't always choose the easy alternative, though—all the recipes here are quick to make and will stop you feeling deprived while you slim (one of the main reasons why dieters fall off the wagon). Remember, if you don't like a particular ingredient, you can swap it for an alternative (see page 25 for further information on how to do this).

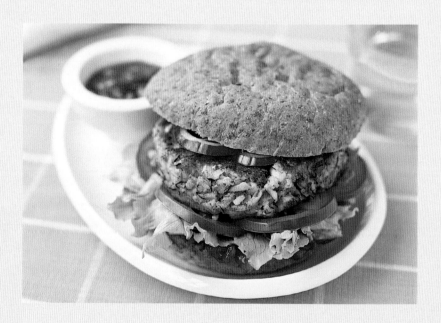

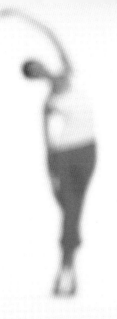

feel good

The "feel good" tips aim either to enhance the weight-loss effects of the diet or, simply, to create a healthier, happier body to show off your new shape. Again, adding a tip each day (or at least two or three times a week) will boost your results and/or your all-round health. You don't have to follow the tips in the order in which they appear; you can try them in whatever order best fits your mood or personal needs.

fit

On pages 90–103 you'll find an easy ten-minute exercise plan to carry out each day. This helps to tone and strengthen your muscles and will enhance the weight-loss effects of the diet. Each day on the 14-day plan you'll also find a suggestion for a "fit" task. This will help to increase the calories that you burn each day, and you should aim to add at least two of these tasks each week (or, even better, try a new one each day). Remember, the amount of weight you lose on any diet is determined by the difference between the number of calories you eat and the number you burn off. You'll find some extra exercise suggestions on pages 104–107. To really boost results, aim for 30–60 minutes of any of these at least two or three times a week.

socializing on the plan

One of the biggest problems when following a diet is that life can often get in the way. Eating out or having friends round for dinner may appear to be difficult, but as long as you stick to some simple rules, it really needn't be a problem.

• Eat low-calorie and low-GI, whatever happens. If you're going out for dinner, stick to two courses and make sensible low-calorie choices. Good appetizer suggestions are clear soups, smoked salmon or shrimp cocktail, chicken tikka or prosciutto with melon. For the main course, choose plain fish, meat or poultry with salad (carbs are best avoided) or a small portion of pasta with a fish or vegetable sauce. Most desserts tend to be high in GI or calories, so skip these if possible or order a small scoop of ice cream or sorbet. It might not be your dream order, but the plan is only for 14 days.

• Avoid alcohol altogether as it increases your appetite and boosts fluid retention.

• If you're cooking for other people, swap the evening meal for one of the more exotic suggestions, such as Lemon and Lime Chicken (page 85), Gingered Salmon (page 45), or Spicy Beef (page 69). The calorie count may differ slightly from your recommended meal, but it will still be low-GI enough to get results. Afterwards serve a low-calorie dessert, such as the jelly on page 33, or some fresh figs with a little crème fraîche.

Getting started

It's a lot easier to stick to a plan if you've got the ingredients you need for each day in your pantry. Below you'll find a simple shopping list of things you might need to stock up on before you start the plan. Opposite are the answers to some questions that might be going through your head right now.

diet shopping list

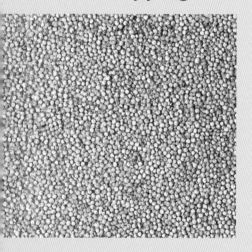

• **Seeds and nuts:** if you find these irresistible, divide them into small handful-size packs covered with plastic wrap.

• **Herbs and spices used in the recipes:** most of these are common herbs like basil or mint, but do check that you have everything you need.

• **Sourdough/soy linseed bread:** you'll find these on the bread counter at large supermarkets or in health-food stores. If you can't find them, multigrain bread is an alternative.

• **Spelt crisp breads:** these are made of a particularly low-GI type of flour. Again, you'll find them in health-food stores or in the specialty foods section of your local supermarket. Rye crisp breads or oatcakes make good replacements.

• **Canned beans or lentils:** these are a quick-fix alternative to using legumes that need to be soaked before cooking. To determine your portion size, as a general rule, use a quantity three times that of the dry amount suggested in any recipe.

• **Grains such as bulgar and quinoa:** these are lower GI alternatives to rice or couscous, and you'll find them in health-food stores or supermarkets. Quinoa is the quickest to cook (taking 15 minutes), while bulgar needs to be soaked for about 30 minutes.

• **Low-GI breakfast cereals,** such as noodle-shaped bran varieties, low-sugar granola, and rolled oats: there are many different recipes on offer for breakfast, but if you're pushed for time in the morning it's ok to start the day with 3 tablespoons cereal (½ cup oats), topped or made up with ⅔ cup skim milk and a piece of fruit. Remember, breakfast is the most important meal of the day!

what if I'm vegetarian?

If you're vegetarian there's always an option in the plan for you. In addition, you can adapt any of the recipes by replacing the meat in them with a vegetarian alternative such as tofu, tempeh, TVP, beans or legumes or just a selection of vegetables. In most cases this will lower the calorie count as well, so use 50 percent more than the amount suggested in the recipe to prevent you from eating too little each day.

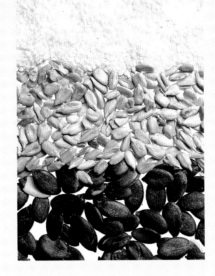

what if I work all day?

While most of the meal options for lunch can easily be taken to work (or, in many cases, bought from the supermarket or local salad bar on the day), if you really don't have time to make complicated lunches or have only limited resources near your workplace, here are three simple low-GI lunches that you can eat on any day and know that you won't bust your calorie budget.

• Two slices of multigrain bread spread with a little mustard and filled with two or three slices of ham, chicken, roast beef, or 2 tablespoons tuna in brine. Add unlimited salad and serve with a small can of slimmer's soup or with three handfuls of baby carrots or celery sticks.

• One small (tennis-ball-size) baked potato, topped with 3 tablespoons baked beans. Follow this with a piece of fruit.

• A salad made from a mix of any vegetables you like and topped with three slices of ham, chicken, or roast beef, 1 oz low-fat cheese, ⅓ cup low-fat cottage cheese, or 2 oz tuna and two crispbreads or oatcakes.

what if I eat my main meal at lunch?

Then swap things round—there's no reason why you can't.

what if I'm a night-time nibbler?

This is a major problem for dieters and one of the reasons why each evening meal of this 14-day plan has a suggested dessert. If you know you like to eat at night, don't eat this immediately after your main meal, but wait until your normal "nibble" time and have it then.

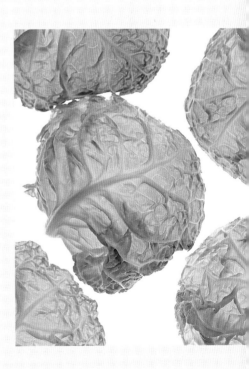

day 1

A new day and a new diet—but this one will be unlike anything you've tried before. There are going to be no hunger pangs, no feelings of deprivation, and no sugar cravings to have you searching for chocolate at 3 p.m. This time losing weight is going to feel simple and satisfying.

food

breakfast

glass of apple juice or unsweetened cranberry juice
⅔ cup

toast with jelly
Spread sugar-reduced jelly thinly on 2 slices of toasted sourdough, soy/linseed, or multigrain bread.

ALTERNATIVE
bowl of bran cereal or low-sugar granola
3 tablespoons cereal with ¾ cup skim milk.

snack

carton of low-fat yogurt with strawberries or raspberries
½ cup plain yogurt served with a handful of strawberries or raspberries.

lunch

baked potato, baked beans, and salad
Top a large baked potato (8 oz) with 5 tablespoons baked beans. Serve with a large green salad made with cucumber, lettuce, and assorted salad leaves.

ALTERNATIVE
broiled tomatoes and mushrooms
Serve on 2 slices of toasted sourdough, soy/linseed, or multigrain bread.

dessert

apple

snack

handful of peanuts and raisins
3 tablespoons

dinner

low-GI vegetable stir-fry
(see page 32)

ALTERNATIVE
broiled ham steak with vegetables
Broil a 4 oz ham steak and serve with 2 small sweet potatoes, mashed with a little garlic and skim milk, and a large portion of snow peas and carrots.

dessert

real strawberry Jello
(see page 33)

fit

Burning calories each day needn't be tricky. Recent research from the Mayo Clinic in the United States revealed that the difference between naturally thin people and those who tend to put on weight is something called the NEAT factor. NEAT stands for Non Exercise Achieved Thermogenesis —and in simple terms it means that the more you walk, stand, or fidget each day, the more calories you burn and the thinner you're likely to be.

Up your NEAT factor each day by standing or pacing to make phone calls, by always taking the stairs or walking up the escalator, and by doing all those things your parents told you not to do, such as tapping your fingers or feet as you sit. Remember, every single move you make each day burns calories.

feel good

Each day of the 14-day diet plan you can have ¾ cup of skim or low-fat milk for use in teas and coffees. In addition, you should aim to drink at least 8 cups of water each day—that's between six and eight glasses. This isn't just to stop you feeling thirsty; when you're dehydrated, your metabolism slows down by as much as 3 percent, which means you will burn up to 60 fewer calories a day, which adds up to 6 pounds a year in weight that you could have lost.

To boost your fluid intake, drink either tap or bottled water. If you don't like the taste of water, put a splash of fruit juice or low-sugar cordial or concentrate in it to flavor it. Or try herbal teas, either drunk hot or mixed in a large pitcher and cooled in the refrigerator—this works really well with fruit teas such as blackberry or with a cooling peppermint blend.

Alcohol doesn't count towards your 8 cups each day as it dehydrates the body, adds calories, and reduces your levels of vital fat-burning B vitamins. Caffeine has a similar effect, so try to stick to fewer than four cups of tea or coffee a day, or choose decaffeinated blends.

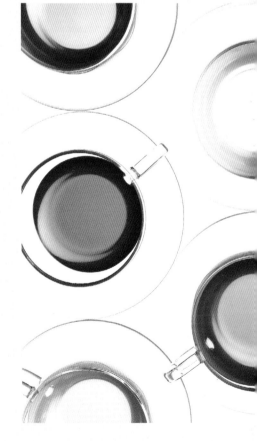

low-GI vegetable stir-fry

preparation: 10 minutes | **cooking:** 20 minutes | **serves:** 4

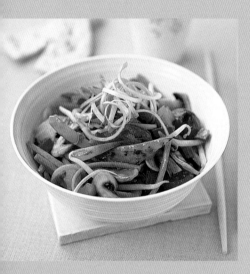

1 tablespoon olive oil or canola oil

1 large onion, diced

1 large red bell pepper, cored, seeded, and diced

2 celery sticks, sliced

2 tablespoons light soy sauce

2 tablespoons tomato ketchup

pinch of chili powder

4 oz mushrooms, trimmed and sliced

10 cherry tomatoes, halved

4 oz snow peas or green beans, halved if large

2 cups bean sprouts

2 large carrots, cut into batons

4 whole-wheat pita breads, to serve

scallion curls, to garnish (optional)

1 Heat the oil in a large nonstick pan or wok. Add the onion and cook for 2 minutes.

2 Add the bell pepper and celery and sauté for a few minutes. Add the soy sauce, tomato ketchup, and chili powder and stir well.

3 Add the remaining vegetables and stir-fry over a medium heat for 10–15 minutes until the vegetables are tender. Add a small amount of water if necessary.

4 Garnish the stir-fry with scallion curls, if desired, and accompany each serving with a whole-wheat pita bread.

nutritional values per serving
Kcals **121 (508 kJ)**
Protein **5.5 g**
Carb **17.2 g**
Sodium **44 mg**
Fat **3.8 g**
Sat. fat **0.6 g**
GI **Low**

tip

This recipe can be easily adapted to a different selection of vegetables. If you need to eat it in a hurry, serve in a pita pocket or a tortilla.

real strawberry Jello

preparation: 5 minutes | **chilling time:** 1–2 hours | **serves:** 4

1 package (about ½ oz) sugar-free strawberry Jello gelatin

1 cup strawberries, hulled, and sliced if large

strawberries, to decorate

low-fat cream, to serve

1 Make up the Jello according to the instructions on the package.

2 Arrange the strawberries in a mold or basin. Slowly pour the Jello into the mold. Chill for 1–2 hours or until firmly set.

3 To turn out the Jello from a mold, dip the base of the mould in a bowl of hot water for about 10 seconds. Loosen the edge of the Jello with a fingertip and invert a serving plate on top of the mold. Turn upside down and shake firmly—the Jello should be released. If not, re-dip the mold in hot water and repeat. If the Jello is made in a basin, run a knife around the side and then invert onto a plate and shake firmly.

4 Decorate with more strawberries and serve with a drizzle of low-fat cream.

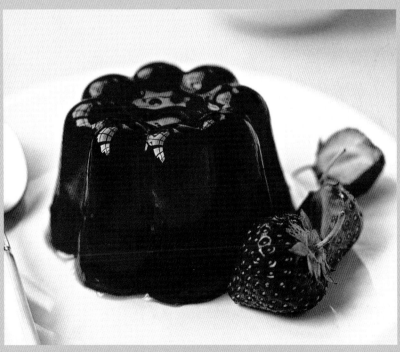

nutritional values per serving
Kcals **20 (84 kJ)**
Protein **2.2 g**
Carb **2.5 g**
Sodium **71 mg**
Fat **0 g**
Sat. fat **0 g**
GI **Low**

day 2

If you didn't weigh yourself yesterday, get on the scales first thing this morning. Your body's weight-loss systems will already have started to burn fat, while all the extra water you're drinking will ensure that any excess fluid is beginning to be released from your tissues—and you'll want to measure your progress from the outset to get the most motivational results.

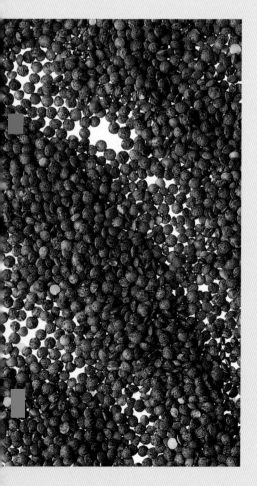

food

breakfast

bowl of porridge
Made using 3 tablespoons rolled oats and ¾ cup water or skim milk. Top with a handful of strawberries or raspberries.

ALTERNATIVE
toast and peanut butter
Spread peanut butter on 2 slices of toasted sourdough, soy/linseed, or multigrain bread.

snack

pear

lunch

low-GI lentil and zucchini soup
(see page 36)

ALTERNATIVE
bought sandwich
Choose a sandwich made with multigrain bread and with fewer than 300 kcals.

dessert

slice of melon or handful of berries

snack

carton of low-fat plain yogurt
½ cup

dinner

blackened cod with citrus salsa
(see page 37)

ALTERNATIVE
omelet
Made with 2 eggs and cooked in a nonstick pan with a minimum of canola or olive oil. Fill with mushrooms, onions, and zucchini or 2 slices of lean ham. Serve with a large green side salad and a multigrain roll.

dessert

fresh fruit salad
Made with a selection of fruit, such as a sliced banana, sliced apple, orange and grapefruit segments, and strawberries, with a little added unsweetened orange juice.

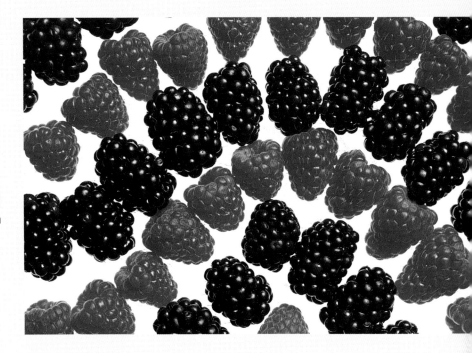

fit

Dancing is a great way to burn calories—and, because it's fun, you don't always notice how long you're "exercising" for. Research at Springfield College, Massachusetts, has discovered that exercisers work out on average 27 percent longer if they do it to music. So, close the curtains, put on your favorite CD and dance around the house for 30 minutes.

feel good

Stress can affect your waistline. Not only does feeling under pressure make it more likely that you'll comfort-eat, but stress hormones such as cortisol actually contribute to fat storage —especially in the tummy area. One of the easiest ways to unwind is in an aromatherapy bath. Lavender is the most commonly used aromatherapy oil, but there are other essential oils that can help dieters boost their motivation.

Try making a blend of two drops of thyme, rosemary, and grapefruit (added to 1 teaspoon carrier oil) to boost your motivation and feelings of success; or use two drops of frankincense plus two of lavender to give you a great night's sleep, thereby preventing fatigue-related nibbles the next day. So turn on the faucets, add your aromatherapy oil as the bath runs to enhance the scents, shut the door and indulge in half an hour of serenity and calm.

fact

People who follow a low-GI diet tend to have lower blood pressure than those who eat the high-GI way.

low-GI lentil and zucchini soup

preparation: 10 minutes | **cooking:** 45 minutes | **serves:** 4

2 vegetable bouillon cubes

2 cups boiling water

¼ cup lentils

4 zucchini, chopped

4 small onions, chopped

13 oz can chopped tomatoes

1 teaspoon chopped fresh mixed herbs

pepper

4 multigrain rolls, to serve

1 Dissolve the bouillon cubes in the boiling water in a saucepan. Add the lentils and simmer for 15 minutes.

2 Add all the remaining ingredients to the pan and cook for 30 minutes or until the vegetables are soft

3 Keep the soup chunky by briefly crushing the vegetables with a potato crusher. Serve immediately with multigrain rolls.

tip

This is a really substantial soup and easy to cook. If you have not made soup before it will inspire you to make other soups using a different selection of vegetables. The soup can easily be transported in a flask for a packed lunch.

nutritional values per serving
Kcals **110 (465 kJ)**
Protein **7.0 g**
Carb **18.9 g**
Sodium **633 mg**
Fat **1.5 g**
Sat. fat **0 g**
GI **Low**

blackened cod with citrus salsa

preparation: 10 minutes | **cooking:** 13 minutes | **serves:** 4

1 large orange

1 garlic clove, crushed

2 large tomatoes, seeded and diced

2 tablespoons chopped basil

⅓ cup black olives, chopped

1 tablespoon extra virgin olive oil

4 cod fillets, about 5 oz each

1 tablespoon jerk seasoning

pepper

chopped basil, to garnish

large green salad and 7 oz new potatoes, boiled in their skins, to serve

1 Cut the skin and white membrane from the orange. Working over a bowl to catch the juice, cut between the membranes to remove the segments. Halve the segments and mix them with the reserved orange juice, the garlic, tomatoes, basil, olives, and half the oil. Season with pepper and set aside to infuse as a salsa.

2 Brush the cod fillets with the remaining oil and coat with the jerk seasoning. Heat a large ovenproof pan and fry the cod fillets, skin side down, for 5 minutes. Turn them over and cook them for an additional 3 minutes. Transfer to a preheated oven, 300°F, for about 5 minutes.

3 Garnish the fish with chopped basil and serve with the salsa, a green salad, and new potatoes.

nutritional values per serving
Kcals **216 (904 kJ)**
Protein **28.8 g**
Carb **7.0 g**
Sodium **381 mg**
Fat **8.2 g**
Sat. fat **1.2 g**
GI **Low**

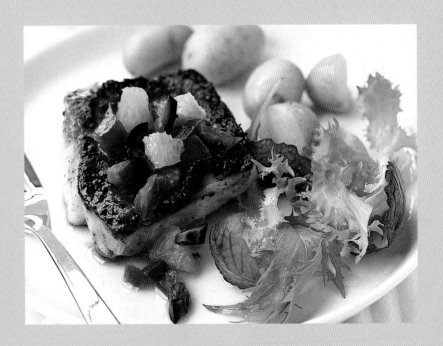

day 3

You should be feeling really positive about this plan now you've realized how easy it is, after all. But from today you'll start to see some extra benefits. Already your blood-sugar levels will have stabilized dramatically, leaving you bursting with vitality. Say goodbye to 3 p.m. energy slumps and hello to a brighter new you.

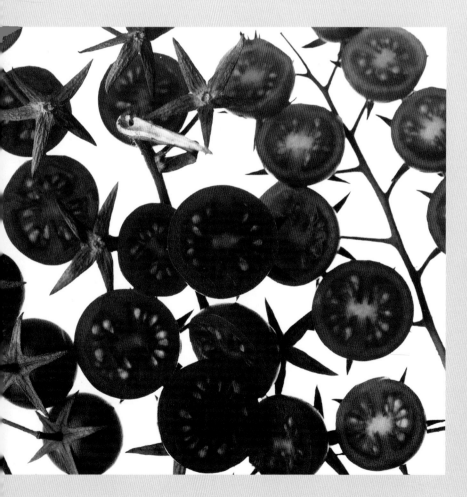

food

breakfast

berry breakfast
(see page 40)

ALTERNATIVE
large pink grapefruit plus 1 slice of toast
Toast 1 slice of multigrain, soy/linseed, or sourdough bread and serve with a scraping of low-fat spread.

snack

2 seeded crisp breads topped with slices of pear or apple

lunch

it's a wrap
(see page 41)

ALTERNATIVE

salad

Made with lettuce and assorted salad leaves, cucumber, grated carrot, plum tomatoes, and radishes together with ⅓ cup low-fat grated cheese or 2 oz lean ham. Serve with a slice of soy and linseed bread.

dessert

banana

snack

low-fat chocolate mousse
Small pot (½ cup) bought from a store or supermarket.

dinner

mixed grill
2 low-fat or vegetarian sausages broiled with large mushrooms and tomatoes and served with 2 small oven-baked sweet potatoes. Accompany with a tomato salsa.

ALTERNATIVE

spaghetti bolognese
Made with 3 oz lean ground beef or 4 oz ground soy per portion with a jar of ready-made tomato sauce and extra mushrooms and onion added. Serve with 2 oz spaghetti per person.

dessert

fresh pineapple slices

fit

It's been estimated by *Prima* magazine that our grandmothers burned three times as many calories each day as we do, because they didn't use any labor-saving gadgets. So at least once a day aim to do a task by hand, instead of using an appliance to do it: easy examples include switching television channels over by hand instead of using the remote (don't laugh; after all, every 20 steps you take walking to the television and back burns a calorie) or washing dishes instead of using the dishwasher.

The ultimate workout, however, is washing the car yourself instead of taking it to the car wash—you'll burn roughly 200 calories in half an hour and give your arms a great workout.

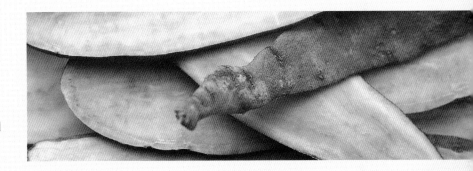

feel good

Smile—it's been proved that your body can't tell the difference between a real smile and a fake one; simply the action of forcing your face into a grin causes mood-boosting endorphin chemicals to be released in the brain. If a low mood gets you down today (and potentially reaching for some sweet treats) stand in front of the mirror and just smile for a few minutes. Your mood will lift immediately.

fact

Many of us don't like berries such as raspberries because of the masses of tiny pips they contain. However, those pips have high levels of a vital natural chemical called ellagic acid. These have been shown to cause cancer cells to self-destruct.

berry breakfast

preparation: 15 minutes plus chilling | **serves:** 4

¼ **cup low-fat Greek yogurt**

2 tablespoons honey

3 cups raspberries

¼ **cup rolled oats**

1 Put the yogurt in a large bowl. Add the honey and fold in.

2 Divide one-third of the raspberries among 4 serving glasses. Cover with half the yogurt mixture. Scatter over some of the oats and more raspberries, dividing them among the glasses.

3 Repeat the layers, finishing with oats and a few raspberries. Chill in the refrigerator for 30 minutes before serving.

tip

This recipe is also great for a dessert. It can easily be varied using different fruits.

nutritional values per serving
kcals **105 (445 kJ)**
Protein **1.8 g**
Carb **22.0 g**
Sodium **16 mg**
Fat **1.5 g**
Sat. fat **0.9 g**
GI **Low**

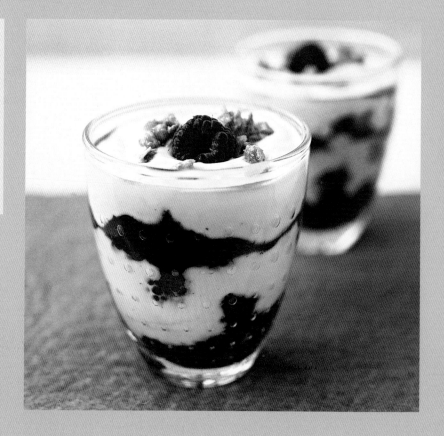

it's a wrap

preparation: 5 minutes | **cooking:** 8–10 minutes | **serves:** 4

1 teaspoon olive oil

2 garlic cloves, finely chopped

1 onion, finely chopped

8 oz lean lamb stir-fry strips, cut small or halved

4 oz mushrooms, finely chopped

1 small red bell pepper, cored, seeded, and sliced

2 tablespoons chopped fresh parsley

2 tablespoons chopped fresh mint

⅔ cup cooked basmati rice

juice of 1 lemon

4 tablespoons low-fat Greek yogurt

2 tablespoons mint sauce

8 flour tortillas or flatbreads

¼ cucumber, cut into strips

arugula salad, to serve

1 To make the filling, heat the oil in a nonstick wok or pan and cook the garlic, onion, and lamb strips for 3–4 minutes until brown. Add the mushrooms and bell pepper and cook for 2–3 minutes. Stir in the herbs, rice, and lemon juice. Heat for an additional 1–2 minutes.

2 Mix together the yogurt and mint sauce.

3 To assemble the wraps, place the flour tortillas on a clean work surface. Spread some of the yogurt mixture over each tortilla, top with a large spoonful of the filling and a few strips of cucumber.

4 Fold up to make a neat roll and serve immediately with an arugula salad.

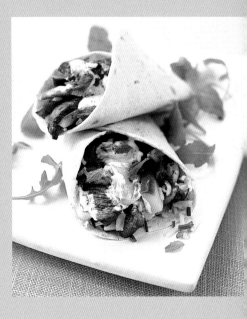

nutritional values per serving
Kcals **408 (1723 kJ)**
Protein **25 g**
Carb **64.2 g**
Sodium **341 mg**
Fat **7.2 g**
Sat. fat **2.4 g**
GI **Low**

tip

Lean lamb is used here but other meat, such as pork, beef, or chicken stir-fry strips, could be substituted. Try chickpeas for a vegetarian alternative.

day 4

By now you should be realizing how easy it is to fit low-GI eating into your daily life. Even if you're trying to combine losing weight with working in an office all day, these quick and easy meals make sticking to things ultra-simple. And almost all the lunches suggested here can easily be made in advance and taken to work from home.

food

breakfast

glass of unsweetened orange juice
⅓ cup

broiled mushrooms on toast
Broil 2 large mushrooms and serve on 2 slices of toasted sourdough, soy/linseed, or multigrain bread.

ALTERNATIVE
breakfast shake
Made by blending together a banana, ⅓ cup skim milk, and 1 tablespoon rolled oats.

snack

nectarine

lunch

chicken and endive salad with sesame seed dressing
(see page 44)

ALTERNATIVE
can or carton of low-calorie vegetable soup
Serve with a large multigrain roll.

dessert

carton of low-fat yogurt with cherries
½ cup plain yogurt, topped with a few cherries.

snack

large apple

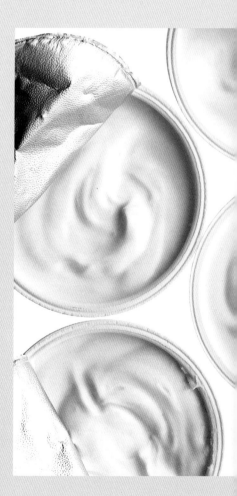

dinner

gingered salmon

(see page 45)

ALTERNATIVE

quinoa and roasted vegetables

Cook ½ cup quinoa or bulgur wheat per person according to the directions on the package. Roast eggplant, zucchini, red and green bell peppers in a spoonful of olive oil. Sprinkle with lemon juice and chopped herbs and serve on top of the quinoa or bulgur wheat.

dessert

raspberry blancmange

Make up 1 portion per person according to the instructions on the package, using skim milk.

fit

Many of us think running is only for the super-fit, but if you're already a regular walker, there's no reason you shouldn't start thinking about incorporating some light jogging into your daily workout (you'll burn twice as many calories per minute if you do).

The best way to get started is to alternate 30-second or one-minute bursts of jogging with four minutes of walking. If you're asked how hard you're working on a scale of ten, a sensible pace should feel like about seven or eight. As you get fitter, your jogging breaks can get longer and your walking breaks shorter. Next thing you know, you're a runner!

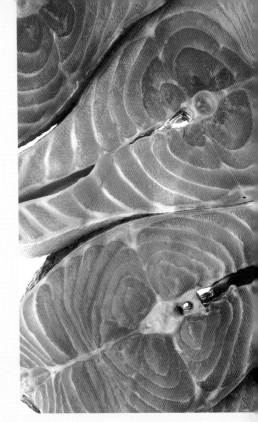

feel good

Doing something that absorbs your mind not only prevents you from snacking out of boredom but research is showing that it can boost your immune system and exercise your brain in a way that actually triggers it to create new cells (something that may help prevent age-related memory problems). Instead of slumping in front of the television each night, try to do something engaging tonight. If you're a creative type, get out some paints; if you're a fashionista, you may want to take up knitting; or just buy yourself a jigsaw and pick up those pieces. You'll be amazed how time will fly.

fact

Sunlight could make you slim. The action of sunlight on your skin produces vitamin D—and without this you absorb only 10 percent of the calcium you take in (with it, this increases to 80–90 percent). That is bad news for dieters, as recent research has revealed that calcium turns fat-storing cells into fat-burning ones! So aim to get outside for 30 minutes a day to boost your vitamin D levels.

chicken and endive salad with sesame seed dressing

preparation: 20 minutes | **serves:** 4

2 oz lettuce, torn into pieces

2 heads Belgian endive, sliced

¼ cucumber, diced

2 oz broccoli florets, cooked

2 large pink grapefruit, peeled and segmented

4 oz roast chicken, cut into strips

13 oz can chickpeas, drained

1 large yellow bell pepper, cored, seeded, and sliced

1 large green bell pepper, cored, seeded, and sliced

1 cup cherry tomatoes, halved

4 slices grain and linseed bread

Dressing

½ teaspoon sugar

½ tablespoon Dijon mustard

2 tablespoons white wine vinegar

2 tablespoons olive oil

½ tablespoon sesame seeds

1 tablespoon soy sauce, optional

pepper

1 Toss the lettuce, endive, cucumber, broccoli, and grapefruit in a bowl.

2 Add the chicken, chickpeas, bell peppers, and tomatoes.

3 For the dressing mix the sugar, mustard, and vinegar and beat. Drizzle in the oil while still beating then add the pepper.

4 Dry-fry the sesame seeds until lightly browned then toss with the soy sauce, if desired, and quickly cover with a lid. When cool, add to the dressing.

5 Add the dressing to the salad and serve the salad with slices of grain and linseed bread.

nutritional values per serving
Kcals **188 (794 kJ)**
Protein **16.8 g**
Carb **23.8 g**
Sodium **167 mg**
Fat **4.0 g**
Sat. fat **0.7 g**
GI **Low**

tip

Endive gives a wonderful flavor but if you cannot find it use romaine lettuce or bok choy. If you do not eat chicken you could make this recipe with tofu, nuts, or extra chickpeas.

gingered salmon

preparation: 10 minutes | **cooking:** 6–10 minutes | **serves:** 4

½ **bunch scallions, shredded**

1 inch piece of fresh ginger root, peeled and cut into strips

2 tablespoons low-calorie American dry ginger ale or made-up low-calorie ginger cordial

2 tablespoons light soy sauce

4 salmon fillets, about 4 oz each without skin

cabbage, snow peas, and 7 oz new potatoes, boiled in their skins, to serve

1 Mix the scallions, fresh ginger, ginger ale or cordial, and soy sauce in a bowl.

2 Place the salmon in a covered skillet and poach in the mixture for 3–5 minute each side. Top up with a little water if needed.

3 Serve with steamed cabbage, snow peas, and new potatoes. Garnish with the scallions and ginger and pour over a little of the ginger ale mixture.

nutritional values per serving
Kcals **233 (971 kJ)**
Protein **25.8 g**
Carb **1.3 g**
Sodium **57 mg**
Fat **13.8 g**
Sat. fat **2.4 g**
GI **Low**

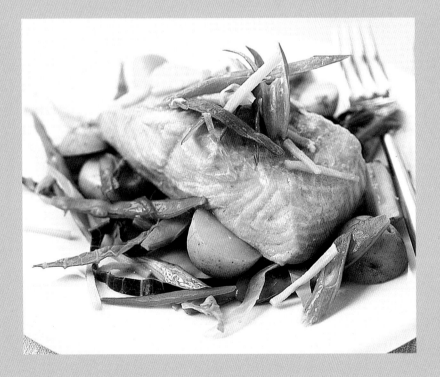

day 5

You may not have realized it, but every day so far on this plan you've reached your recommended daily intake of five portions of fruit and vegetables. This was recently announced as one of the main healthy habits that lead to sustained weight loss, so it's great news for your diet—and vital for all-round well-being.

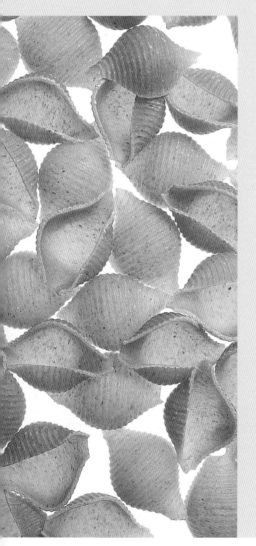

food

breakfast

bowl of soy and linseed cereal
Use 3 tablespoons cereal with ⅓ cup skim milk. Top with a sliced small banana.

ALTERNATIVE
toast with peanut butter
Spread 1 teaspoon peanut butter on 2 slices of toasted sourdough, soy/linseed, or multigrain bread.

snack

1 oat biscuit with a thin scraping of low-fat soft cheese

lunch

pasta with lentil and bell pepper sauce
(see page 48)

ALTERNATIVE
small carton of low-fat hummus and crudités
½ cup hummus served with raw carrots, celery, and cauliflower florets and 4 seeded rye crisp breads

dessert

2 kiwifruit

snack

low-fat plain yogurt topped with blackberries
½ cup

dinner

romaine lettuce salad with Gorgonzola and walnuts
(see page 49)

Serve with oven-baked potato wedges made by slicing 1 large baking potato (6 oz) per person, into slender wedges, drizzling with some soy sauce and baking for approximately 20 minutes at the top of a hot oven, 400°F, until crisp.

ALTERNATIVE
chicken salad
Made from a selection of salad leaves, cilantro, sliced tomatoes, and scallions, up to 1 cup drained canned chickpeas, 1 tablespoon pumpkin seeds, and 4 oz sliced broiled chicken breast tossed in 1 tablespoon low-calorie vinaigrette.

dessert

1 large pear

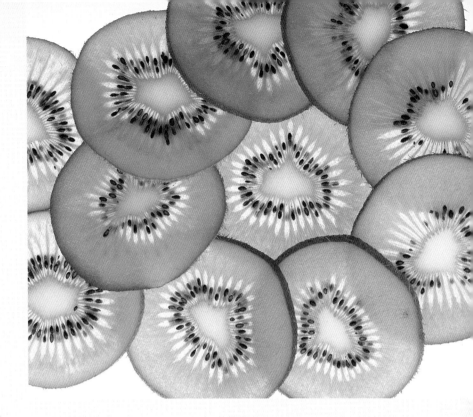

fact

Pears contain the vital mineral iodine, which helps to maximize thyroid function. As the thyroid is the gland that controls how many calories you burn each day, having it firing on all cylinders is vital for slimming success.

fit

Go swimming. Many of us only ever visit the pool during our summer break, but it's a great all-round body toner and a perfect exercise for those who don't currently work out. Not only does swimming put no pressure on your joints, but your position in the water means that you actually feel less fatigued swimming than exercising in other ways at the same intensity.

If you're not a great swimmer, the pool isn't completely off the exercise schedule for you. Walking—or even running—in water over waist height creates extra resistance, boosting the toning effects of these exercises.

feel good

Take time over your meals today and every day: eating quickly is a common cause of bloating that adds to your waistline. Other belly-boosting activities include chewing gum, talking while eating, and drinking from a sports-top bottle or while exercising—all of which trigger excess gas. If you do suffer, peppermint tea can help reduce the effects.

pasta with lentil and bell pepper sauce

preparation: 15 minutes | **cooking:** 35–40 minutes | **serves:** 4

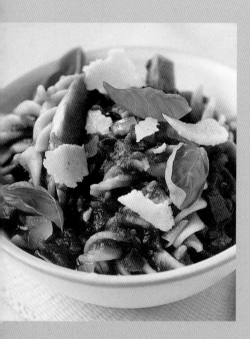

½ cup split red lentils

1 tablespoon olive oil

2 onions, chopped

2 small red bell peppers, cored, seeded, and chopped

4 large mushrooms, trimmed and sliced

1 garlic clove, crushed

2 tablespoons chopped fresh basil, plus extra to garnish

2 tablespoons chopped fresh oregano or parsley

13 oz can tomatoes

2 tablespoons tomato paste

1 cup water

pinch of sugar

8 oz whole-wheat pasta

pepper

grated Parmesan cheese, to serve

1 Boil the lentils in water for 15 minutes. Drain.

2 Heat the oil in a nonstick pan and fry the onions and bell peppers for 10 minutes. Add the lentils, mushrooms, garlic, herbs, tomatoes, tomato paste, water, sugar, and pepper.

3 Bring to a boil then turn down the heat and simmer gently, uncovered, for 15–20 minutes.

4 15 minutes before the sauce is ready half-fill a saucepan with water and bring to a boil. Add the pasta and boil rapidly for 10–12 minutes, or according to the instructions on the package, until the pasta is cooked. Drain.

5 Garnish with fresh basil leaves and serve with grated Parmesan.

nutritional values per serving
Kcals **391 (1659 kJ)**
Protein **19.2 g**
Carb **71.4 g**
Sodium **162 mg**
Fat **5.3 g**
Sat. fat **0.7 g**
GI **Low**

romaine lettuce salad with Gorgonzola and walnuts

preparation: 10 minutes | **serves:** 4

2 tablespoons olive oil

1 tablespoon good white wine vinegar

4 oz Gorgonzola cheese

1 cup shelled walnuts, coarsely chopped

1 romaine lettuce, torn into bite-size pieces

pepper

potato wedges, to serve

1 Put the oil, vinegar, and a little pepper into a salad bowl and mix thoroughly. Add half the Gorgonzola and mash it well with a fork.

2 Add half the chopped walnuts and all the lettuce, and toss until evenly coated with the dressing.

3 Top with the remaining Gorgonzola, cut into small pieces, and the rest of the chopped walnuts.

nutritional values per serving
Kcals **250 (1050 kJ)**
Protein **9 g**
Carb **1 g**
Sodium **346 mg**
Fat **23 g**
Sat. fat **8 g**
GI **Low**

tip

This really light recipe will serve 8 as a dinner-party appetizer. You can vary the ingredients by using Roquefort instead of Gorgonzola if you prefer a stronger taste.

day 6

If you started this diet on a Monday, it is now the weekend with all the temptations that can occur. However, by kicking off with a hearty breakfast—and finishing the day with a meal that definitely won't make you feel as if you're dieting—you're assured of success.

food

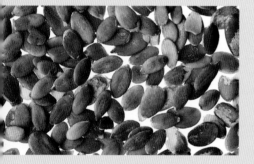

breakfast

kedgeree
(see page 52)

ALTERNATIVE
glass of tropical fruit juice
⅔ cup

carton of low-fat yogurt and raspberries, plus 1 crumpet or English muffin, toasted

snack

mix of seeds and nuts
3 tablespoons

lunch

broiled tomatoes
Serve on 2 slices of toasted sourdough, soy/linseed, or multigrain bread.

ALTERNATIVE
can or carton of low-fat lentil soup
Serve with a multigrain roll.

dessert

2 large plums

snack

1 oat biscuit topped with apple slices

dinner

broiled sirloin steak with couscous, salad leaves, and three-bean salad
(see page 53)
Broil a 4 oz steak. Make up ½ cup couscous according to the instructions on the package and serve with the bean salad and a selection of salad leaves.

ALTERNATIVE
broiled veggie burger
Fill 2 small pita breads with strips of a broiled vegetable burger, grated carrot, couscous made according to the instructions on the package, chopped tomato, and strips of cucumber with chopped mint and a low-fat yogurt dressing.

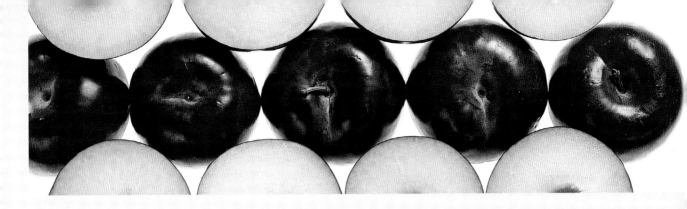

dessert

baked banana and low-fat plain yogurt
Use 1 banana and ½ carton (¼ cup) low-fat plain yogurt. Serve sprinkled with a few chocolate strands.

fit

Skipping is an incredible calorie-burning exercise, using up more than 600 calories an hour, which is equivalent to running at 6 mph. The best thing about it, however, is that it can easily be done in the privacy of your own home—all you need is a skipping rope and some supportive trainers to prevent ankle injuries.

Aim for five minutes today (you may need to do it in one-minute bursts), then build up to 15–20 minutes a day.

feel good

While it's meant to be a break from the working week, the weekend is spent by many of us rushing around even more intensely than usual. If you've got a hectic day ahead, at least spend five minutes relaxing.

A quick meditation technique is to lie down or sit in a chair and gradually relax each part of your body, feeling it grow looser and heavier. Become aware of your breathing and gradually slow it down, so that you carefully decelerate your exhaled breath until it is slower than your inhaled breath. As thoughts enter your head, see them roll up and out of your mind—rather like watching the credits at the end of a movie. After five (or more) minutes, gradually stop the relaxation by gently clenching and then relaxing each muscle of your body, starting from your jaw and moving down to your feet. Now open your eyes and see how refreshed you feel.

fact

The beans that you find in today's three-bean salad are a great source of soluble fibre, which has a beneficial effect in helping to lower blood-cholesterol levels and blood-sugar levels. Other good sources of soluble fibre include oats, peas and lentils.

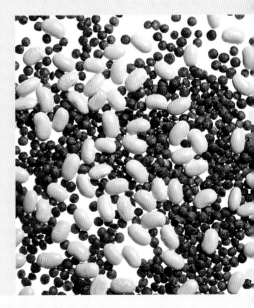

kedgeree

preparation: 10 minutes | **cooking:** 20 minutes | **serves:** 4

8 oz smoked haddock

1¼ cups low-fat coconut milk

½ cup brown lentils

1 teaspoon vegetable oil

1 small onion, chopped finely

4 oz button mushrooms, trimmed and sliced

1 teaspoon tandoori paste

1 cup cooked brown basmati rice

2 hard-cooked eggs, chopped

pepper

cilantro, to garnish

1 Poach the haddock in the coconut milk for 8 minutes and allow to cool. Reserve the milk. Remove the skin from the cooled haddock and flake the flesh.

2 Meanwhile, cook the lentils in boiling water for 15 minutes and drain.

3 Heat the oil and cook the onion for 2 minutes, add the sliced mushrooms and cook for an additional 2 minutes. Add the tandoori paste.

4 Add the rice and lentils to the onion and mushrooms. Add enough of the reserved coconut milk to moisten the mixture and season with pepper. Mix well then add the haddock and eggs.

5 Serve immediately, garnished with a sprig of cilantro.

nutritional values per serving
Kcals **436 (1830 kJ)**
Protein **27.4 g**
Carb **54.5 g**
Sodium **592 mg**
Fat **12.3 g**
Sat. fat **1.0 g**
GI **Low**

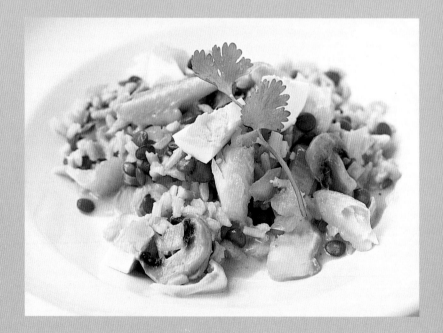

three-bean salad

preparation: 10 minutes | **cooking:** 5 minutes | **serves:** 4

tip

There are endless variations for this easy salad. You can substitute a small can of corn kernals for one of the cans of beans; add other salad vegetables, such as cherry tomatoes, radish slices, cucumber, and grated carrots; or add cooked chicken or flaked tuna. Mix the salad with cooked rice or pasta for a meal on its own.

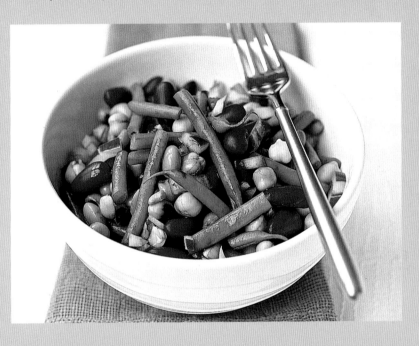

nutritional values per serving
Kcals **212 (898 kJ)**
Protein **14.4 g**
Carb **34.8 g**
Sodium **476 mg**
Fat **2.6 g**
Sat. fat **0.4 g**
GI **Low**

¾ cup sliced green beans

13 oz can red kidney beans, rinsed and drained

13 oz can black-eyed beans, rinsed and drained

13 oz can chickpeas, rinsed and drained

1 small red onion, finely chopped

1 tablespoon balsamic vinegar

1 tablespoon lemon juice

1 Cook the green beans in boiling water for 5 minutes. Drain and then cool by rinsing under a cold tap.

2 Mix the green beans, kidney beans, black-eyed beans, chickpeas, and onion together.

3 Pour over the vinegar and lemon juice and toss to coat evenly. Serve.

day 7

At the end of today you'll be halfway through your diet, and hopefully you've now realized how easy losing weight the GI way can be. If you are having trouble motivating yourself, however, spend a few minutes at the end of the day thinking about all the positive feelings you have experienced this week to encourage you to stick with things next week, too.

food

breakfast

glass of cranberry juice
⅔ cup

bowl of porridge
Use 3 tablespoons rolled oats and make up with water according to the instructions on the package. Serve with ¾ cup skim milk.

ALTERNATIVE
toasted bread with pumpkin seeds and peanut butter, plus two apricots or plums
If you have a bread-maker or make your own bread by hand try adding pumpkin seeds to the mix; if using ready-made bread, toast 2 slices and spread with peanut butter then sprinkle with pumpkin seeds.

snack

slice of melon

lunch

cheesy potato bake
(see page 56)

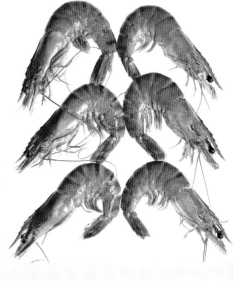

ALTERNATIVE
roast chicken breast

Serve 4 oz chicken breast with a mixture of 6 oz small new potatoes in their skins, chunks of sweet potatoes and butternut squash roasted in 1 teaspoon canola oil, together with boiled carrots and peas. Make gravy with chicken gravy mix and the water in which the vegetables were boiled.

dessert

prune and apricot pudding
(see page 57)

snack

dried berry mix
3 tablespoons

dinner

spicy shrimp, basmati, and ready stir-fried vegetables

Boil basmati rice according to the instructions on the package, allowing ¼ cup per person, and prepare the stir-fried vegetables as directed. Toss 3 oz cooked shrimp, or 5 oz tofu, in 1 teaspoon sweet chili sauce. Pile the rice onto a plate, top with the stir-fried vegetables and shrimp.

ALTERNATIVE
open sandwich

Made with 1 slice of sourdough, soy/linseed, or multigrain bread spread with a thin layer of yeast extract or beef extract and topped with ½ cup cottage cheese, sliced cucumber, tomatoes, and strips of yellow bell pepper.

dessert

2 handfuls fresh cherries
Serve with 2 tablespoons silken tofu or low-fat plain yogurt.

feel good

Spend five minutes today thinking about what you've learned about healthy eating so far on the plan— maybe you're surprised at how small a portion of pasta should be or just how easy it is to eat five portions of fruit and vegetables a day. This "learning" approach to dieting has recently been identified by Yale University researchers as one of the most important factors not only in losing weight—but also in keeping it off.

fit

Make the most of extra time at the weekend and move your workout outside, by taking a hike in the countryside (or at least the local park). Take a friend, your partner, the children, or the dog, and walk briskly for at least an hour. Ideally, you should be walking fast enough to feel a little out of breath, but still able to carry on a conversation—this not only helps pass the time, but also indicates that you're in the maximum fat-burning zone for your body. If you cannot talk and walk at the same time, slow down a little.

fact

Purple fruits are packed with antioxidants, so it's no surprise that prunes, in which all those vital nutrients are condensed during the drying process, have been found to contain the highest level of antioxidants of any fruit.

cheesy potato bake

preparation: 15 minutes | **cooking:** 30 minutes | **serves:** 4

1 tablespoon butter

2 lb potatoes, skins left on, sliced

1 cauliflower, broken into florets

14 oz can lima beans, drained

2½ cups skim milk

cornstarch or thickening granules

2 teaspoons Dijon mustard

garlic clove, cut in half

large pinch of grated nutmeg

1 cup grated low-fat Cheddar cheese

pepper

1 Lightly grease a shallow baking dish with the butter.

2 Boil the potatoes and cauliflower together and simmer gently for 10 minutes or until tender. Add the lima beans to the mixture and simmer for 1 minute. Drain.

3 Make a white sauce with the skim milk and cornstarch and stir in the mustard.

4 Rub the cut sides of the garlic over the inside of the greased baking dish. Put the potatoes, cauliflower, and beans into the dish and pour the white sauce over the top. Sprinkle with the grated nutmeg and pepper.

5 Sprinkle grated cheese over the top of the potatoes. Place under a hot preheated broiler for 5 minutes or until the cheese has melted and the top is crispy and golden brown.

nutritional values per serving
Kcals **460 (1944 kJ)**
Protein **28.0 g**
Carb **69.3 g**
Sodium **1062 mg**
Fat **9.9 g**
Sat. fat **4.4 g**
GI **Low**

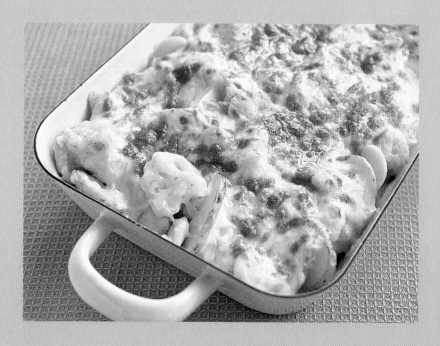

prune and apricot pudding

preparation: 10 minutes | **cooking:** 30–40 minutes | **serves:** 4

¼ cup low-fat spread

¼ cup brown sugar

1 egg, beaten

½ cup self-rising whole-wheat flour

1 tablespoon skim milk

¼ cup ready-to-eat prunes

¼ cup ready-to-eat dried apricots

custard made with skim milk, to serve

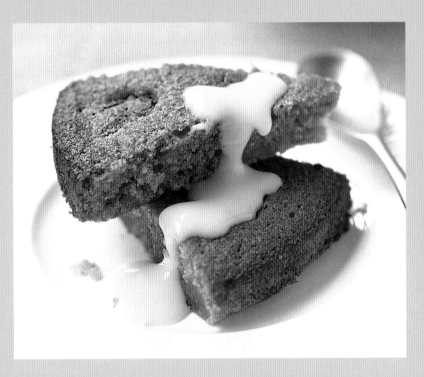

nutritional values per serving
Kcals **197 (829 kJ)**
Protein **4.7 g**
Carb **31.3 g**
Sodium **157 mg**
Fat **6.9 g**
Sat. fat **1.9 g**
GI **Low**

1 Beat together the low-fat spread and sugar until light and fluffy, then add the egg, a little at a time, making sure the egg is well absorbed on each addition. (You can add a little flour with the egg if you wish.) Fold in the remaining flour and add the milk to the mix. It should have a soft dropping consistency.

2 Lightly grease a 7 inch ovenproof dish. Put in a little water and arrange the prunes and apricots over the base.

3 Pour over the pudding mix and spread evenly. Bake in a preheated oven, 350°F, for 30–40 minutes.

4 Serve warm with custard.

day 8

It's the first day of a new week, so when you wake up this morning spend a few minutes repeating to yourself a positive statement, such as "I can stick to this plan again this week" or "I am going to make healthy choices today." This switches on the goal-orientated part of your brain and actively helps you focus on your aims more easily.

food

breakfast

glass of orange juice
⅔ cup

whole-grain bagel with low-fat soft cheese
Spread low-fat soft or cottage cheese thinly on
1 whole-grain bagel.

ALTERNATIVE
bowl of grain or bran cereal
3 tablespoons cereal with
¾ pint skim milk.

snack

handful of gooseberries or greengages, in season, or 1 pear

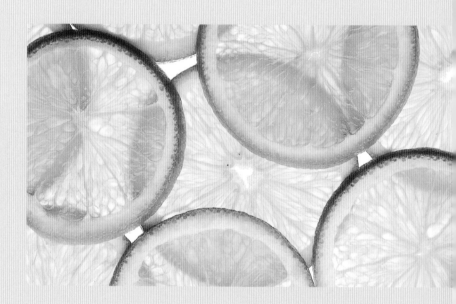

lunch

toasted peanut and wild rice salad
(see page 60)

ALTERNATIVE
spicy sausage and pasta salad
(see page 61)

dessert

frozen yogurt
½ cup

snack

pumpkin seeds
3 tablespoons

dinner

trout with vegetables

Cook 4 oz trout fillet according to the instructions on the pack and serve with steamed snow peas and broccoli and 2 oz boiled potatoes mashed with ½ well-cooked parsnip and 4 tablespoons chickpeas.

ALTERNATIVE

spicy vegetable burger

Broil 4 oz spicy vegetable burger and serve with 2 oz boiled potatoes mashed with ½ well-cooked parsnip and 4 tablespoons chickpeas, plus mushy peas made from a pack of quick-cooked dried peas and gravy.

dessert

cream Jello

Make sugar-free Jello according to the package instructions but use all or a proportion of skim milk instead of water.

fact

Seasonal fruit such as greengages is a great way to liven up your diet. It may also discourage overeating. According to the American Dietetic Association, we don't tend to overeat unfamiliar foods, so experimenting could actually make you thinner.

fit

Every day this week choose one place that you would normally drive to (or take public transport to) and do the same errand on foot, on bike, or even on skates, if you're that way inclined. It might be driving to pick up the morning paper, getting the bus to the station, nipping to get that carton of milk you've forgotten, or heading to a doctor's appointment at lunchtime.

In future try making it a rule for yourself that any journey that would take less than five minutes by car or bus will now be carried out by "alternative" transport.

feel good

By now people may have started to notice that you're eating differently—but don't be tempted to tell everyone that you're trying to lose weight. Sometimes it's better to tell people that you're trying to eat more nutritionally for the sake of your health, rather than for your waistline. This prevents them from trying to tempt you with chocolate or candy.

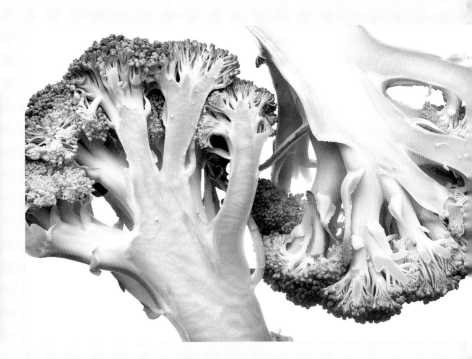

toasted peanut and wild rice salad

preparation: 5 minutes | **cooking:** 30 minutes | **serves:** 4

½ **cup basmati rice**

2 **tablespoons wild rice**

1 **bunch of scallions, chopped**

¾ **cup golden raisins**

¾ **cup toasted peanuts**

4 **tablespoons balsamic vinegar**

1 **tablespoon sunflower oil**

green salad leaves, to serve

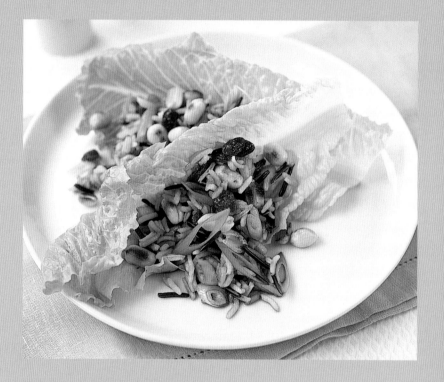

nutritional values per serving
Kcals **427 (1786 kJ)**
Protein **12.0 g**
Carb **56.0 g**
Sodium **8 mg**
Fat **17.5 g**
Sat. fat **3.1 g**
GI **Low**

1 Cook both types of rice according to the instructions on the package then rinse in cold water.

2 Mix the cooked rice, scallions, golden raisins, and peanuts in a large bowl.

3 Pour the vinegar and oil into a small bowl and beat, then stir into the salad.

4 Serve with green salad leaves.

tip

This easy-to-make salad is convenient for picnics and packed lunches and uses stock ingredients. Try adding cucumber, lettuce, and tomatoes too.

spicy sausage and pasta salad

preparation: 10 minutes | **cooking:** 15 minutes | **serves:** 4

tip

This is another easy-to-make salad that's suitable for picnics and packed lunches. The sausages are low in GI—so try different flavors. Vegetarian sausages can also be used, or cooked chicken or hot steak cut into small pieces could be substituted for the sausages.

8 oz whole-wheat pasta spirals

8 low-fat sausages, about 1 lb

1 bunch of scallions

½ head of celery

3 tablespoons low-fat honey and mustard salad dressing

romaine lettuce, to serve

1 Cook the pasta according to the instructions on the package and then rinse in cold water.

2 Prick and then broil the sausages, turning them constantly to reduce the fat content. Drain off the fat and allow the sausages to cool.

3 When cooled, slice the sausages into thick chunks. Cut the scallions and celery into chunks.

4 Mix the pasta, sausages, celery, and scallions with the salad dressing.

5 Serve with romaine lettuce leaves.

nutritional values per serving
Kcals **418 (1763 kJ)**
Protein **23.9 g**
Carb **52.8 g**
Sodium **1074 mg**
Fat **13.9 g**
Sat. fat **4.5 g**
GI **Low**

day 9

You may find that you're getting compliments from other people telling you how well you're looking. This is partly because you have started to lose weight by now, but also because all that water you're drinking—and the high levels of fruit and vegetables, combined with low levels of sugar—means that your skin will have developed a healthy glow.

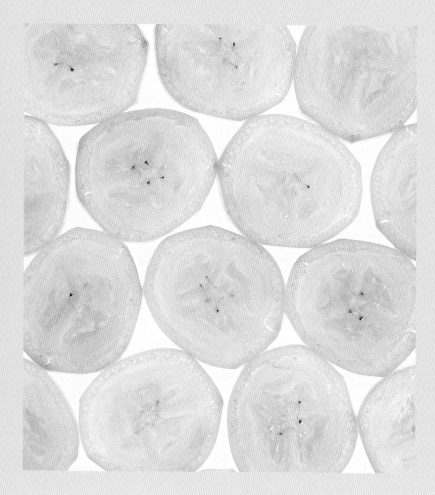

food

breakfast

half a grapefruit

baked beans on sourdough toast
4 tablespoons baked beans on 1 slice of toasted sourdough and flax seed bread.

ALTERNATIVE
multigrain toast with banana
2 slices of toasted multigrain bread topped with a sliced banana.

snack

4 Brazil nuts

lunch

ready-made chicken salad
Accompany a bought ready-made chicken salad (with low-calorie

dressing) with 4 rye multigrain and sunflower seed crisp breads.

ALTERNATIVE
ham and salad sandwich
Made from 2 slices of soy/ linseed bread, lettuce, tomato, and 1 oz lean ham.

dessert

summer pudding
(see page 65)

snack

large nectarine or peach

dinner

cauliflower and chickpea curry
(see page 64)

ALTERNATIVE
salmon fishcakes and spicy fries
Use 2 oz canned salmon per person, mixed with cooked lentils and mashed potatoes and bound together with a beaten egg and rolled in bread crumbs before frying in 1 tablespoon oil. Serve with spicy fries made by sprinkling sticks of sweet potato with soy or chili sauce and oven baking them for about 20 minutes, together with a large green salad.

dessert

melon and raspberries
Cut a slice of melon and serve with raspberries.

fit

Circuit training is a great way to burn calories without getting bored. Build up to being able to repeat the following five exercises four times. You should be working at a rate at which you can speak but not hold a conversation.

1 March on the spot for one minute.

2 Walking lunges: take a large step forward, then lower your hips in a dip. Hold for a second, lift up and take another step.

Repeat, moving back and forth across the room for one minute.

3 Star jumps: standing with your legs hip-width apart, jump up and land with your legs closed; repeat and land with your legs open. Repeat for one minute.

4 Place a ball (or similar small item) on the floor and jump over it from side to side. Repeat for one minute.

5 Walk up and down the stairs for one minute.

feel good

By now sugar cravings should be a thing of the past for you—your blood-sugar levels should be completely under control, although you might find that you still crave sugary treats out of habit at around 3 p.m. If you do, spend a few seconds sitting still, and visualize a rainbow or some roses in your mind. New research from Flinders University in Australia has discovered that this helps stop food cravings in their tracks. This is probably because it takes your mind off them and replaces them with something pleasant, which your mind enjoys thinking about.

fact

Brazil nuts contain high levels of selenium, which acts as an antioxidant and helps the body fight infections and coronary heart disease.

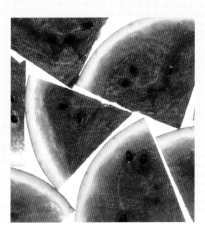

cauliflower and chickpea curry

preparation: 10 minutes | **cooking:** 30 minutes | **serves:** 4

1 tablespoon canola oil

1 large onion, chopped

1–2 garlic cloves, crushed

2 tablespoons medium curry paste

1 cauliflower, cooked and broken into florets

13 oz can chickpeas, drained

2 large potatoes with skins, diced

13 oz can chopped tomatoes

handful of cilantro leaves

basmati rice, to serve

1 Heat the oil in a nonstick pan. Fry the onion and garlic until soft.

2 Add the curry paste and cook for 1 minute.

3 Add the cauliflower, chickpeas, diced potatoes, and tomatoes. Bring to a boil, cover, and simmer for 20–30 minutes until the potatoes are cooked.

4 Remove the lid and boil a few minutes more until the liquid is reduced and thickened. Add the cilantro leaves.

5 Serve with basmati rice.

tip

This is an easy and economical curry to make. If you like your curries really hot add some chili powder. Other vegetables, such as zucchini and mushrooms, can be used in addition to the cauliflower and chickpeas. If you prefer, 4 oz diced cooked lamb or beef can also be added.

nutritional values per serving
Kcals **285 (1201 kJ)**
Protein **13.9 g**
Carb **41.3 g**
Sodium **345 mg**
Fat **8.3 g**
Sat. fat **0.6 g**
GI **Low**

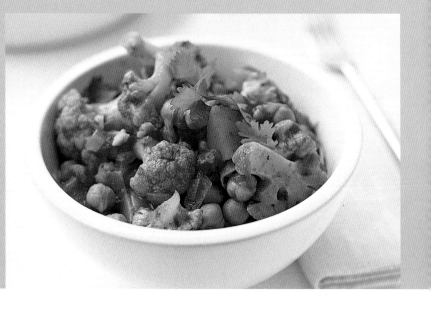

summer pudding

preparation: 30 minutes plus chilling | **cooking:** 10 minutes | **serves:** 4

1 lb mixture of plums, red currants, apples, and raspberries

2 tablespoons superfine sugar

⅓ cup water

6 slices of day-old grain bread

low-fat plain yogurt, to serve

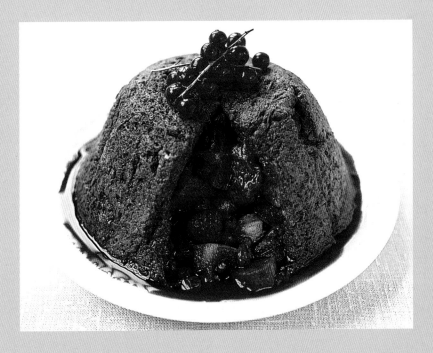

tip

Look out for bargains in late summer when fruit such as plums and damsons are in season and freeze them ready for use in the winter.

nutritional values per serving
Kcals **164 (699 kJ)**
Protein **5.2 g**
Carb **35.2 g**
Sodium **223 mg**
Fat **1.5 g**
Sat. fat **0.2 g**
GI **Low**

1 Put the fruit in a pan with the sugar and the water. Gently heat to a simmer and cook for 10 minutes. Strain the fruit, catching the juice in a bowl.

2 Cut out 2 circles of bread to fit the top and bottom of a 3 cup pudding basin. Shape the rest to fit the sides. Dip the slices in the reserved fruit juice and line the basin.

3 Spoon the fruit into the basin and put the final circle of bread on top. Cover with a saucer and place some cans or weights on top. Chill overnight.

4 Remove the weights and saucer and invert a plate on top. Holding tightly in place, turn the basin over to release the pudding.

5 Serve with low-fat yogurt.

day 10

You're nearing the end of the official two-week plan, and if your willpower is going to fail you, it will be around now, so this morning spend a few minutes looking at yourself in the mirror. Notice any changes, but more importantly focus on any areas of your body that you really like. It's believed this doubles the chance that you'll see a diet out to its end without problems.

food

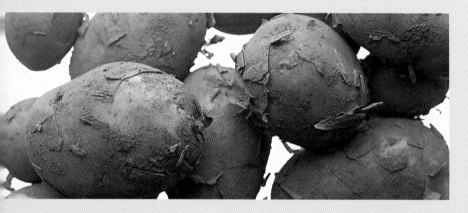

ALTERNATIVE
smoked mackerel with black pepper
4 oz peppered smoked mackerel with a large green salad and a multigrain roll.

dessert

bowl of strawberries with low-fat plain yogurt

breakfast

potato cakes
(see page 68)

ALTERNATIVE
bowl of sugar-free granola
2 tablespoons sugar free granola with ¾ pint skim milk and topped with grated apple.

snack

2 plums

lunch

egg sandwich
Made from 2 slices of multigrain bread filled with a sliced hard-cooked egg, watercress, and 1 teaspoon of light mayonnaise.

snack

low-fat chocolate mousse
Small pot (½ cup) bought from a store or supermarket.

dinner

spicy beef
(see page 69)

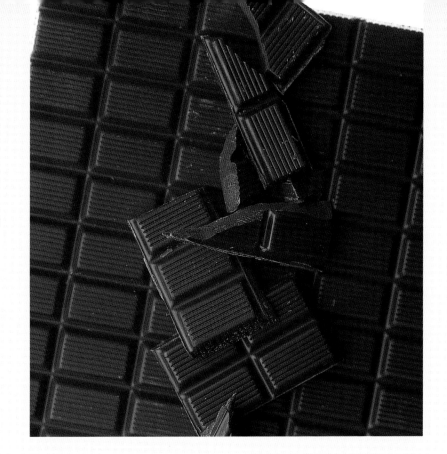

ALTERNATIVE
cauliflower cheese
Use a quarter of a whole cauliflower and a cheese sauce made with 1 oz low-fat cheese and ⅔ cup skim milk thickened with cornstarch. Serve with 1 cup baked beans.

dessert

pineapple and raspberries
2 slices of pineapple canned in its own juice and a handful of raspberries.

fit

Bouncing on a rebounder (a mini-trampoline) isn't just a fun way to burn around 400 calories an hour; it's also believed to be one of the primary ways in which you can increase the activity of the lymph system, which carries waste products out of your body. A stagnant lymph system is one of the contributory causes of cellulite, so if you suffer from this, rebounding may be good exercise to try (weight training is also incredibly effective at fighting cellulite). You'll find rebounders in most sports stores.

feel good

Aim for *lagom* in your life. This Swedish word means "just enough" and harks back to an old Viking tradition whereby people used to bond over a communal cup of mead; they didn't want to take too much or there wouldn't be enough for everyone else. And that's a good way to think about the rest of your life: too much work doesn't leave enough time for family and friends; too many family chores don't leave enough time for you. Think *lagom* in everything you do—including weight loss; in fact, you'll notice that today you get a chocolaty treat to help you do just that.

fact

Beef is an excellent source of iron, which many people (especially women) lack. That's a pity, because low iron levels lead to fatigue—and to a sluggish metabolic rate.

potato cakes

preparation: 10 minutes | **cooking:** 6 minutes | **serves:** 4

1 cup mashed potato

7 oz can corn kernels, drained

2 tablespoons oatbran

1 small egg, lightly beaten

1 tablespoon vegetable oil

tomatoes and mushrooms, to serve

1 Mix the mashed potato, corn, oatbran, and egg in a large bowl. Then divide the mixture into 4 and pat it into flat rounds.

2 Heat the oil in a large nonstick pan and add the cakes one at a time. Cook for 3 minutes then flip over and cook for an additional 3 minutes.

3 Serve with tomatoes and mushrooms.

tip

Potato cakes make a substantial breakfast. They can also be served at other meals and are very good with baked beans.

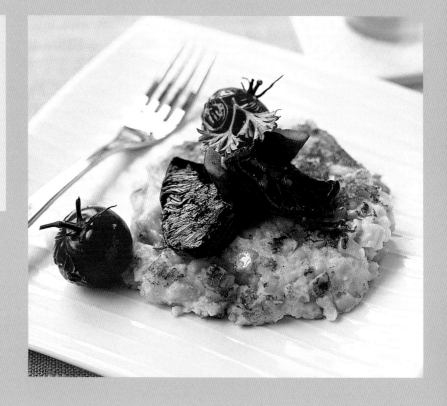

nutritional values per serving
Kcals **148 (621 kJ)**
Protein **4.5 g**
Carb **21.5 g**
Sodium **26 mg**
Fat **5.4 g**
Sat. fat **0.8 g**
GI **Low**

spicy beef

preparation: 10 minutes | **cooking:** 15 minutes | **serves:** 4

1 teaspoon olive oil

1 onion, sliced

1–2 garlic cloves, crushed

1 inch piece of ginger root, peeled and finely chopped

¼ cup all-purpose flour

½ teaspoon turmeric

½ teaspoon chili powder

13 oz beef, cut into strips

1 tablespoon soy sauce

3 tablespoons dry-roasted peanuts

2 cups skim milk

stir-fried vegetables, to serve

1 Heat the oil in a pan and fry the onion, garlic, and ginger for 3–5 minutes. Mix the flour and spices in a bowl and coat the beef, shaking off excess and reserving the rest of the mix.

2 Add the beef to the pan and fry for 3 minutes or until browned.

3 Stir in the reserved flour mix, soy sauce, and peanuts. Cook while stirring for another 2 minutes.

4 Slowly add the milk and stir until the sauce thickens and boils. Cook for 1 minute then cover and simmer for 5 minutes.

5 Serve with stir-fried vegetables.

tip

Beef is a great source of iron. A surprising way to change this dish is to use liver instead of the beef, or try it with pork. The sauce is delicious and really easy to make—the secret is to add the milk slowly. If you want another variation, try using low-fat coconut milk.

nutritional values per serving
Kcals **257 (1078 kJ)**
Protein **27.4 g**
Carb **14.2 g**
Sodium **215 mg**
Fat **10.7 g**
Sat. fat **2.6 g**
GI **Low**

day 11

Yesterday's chocolate treat should have encouraged you a little, but another great trick to try today is to put on a pair of jeans (or other item of clothing) that normally feels a little snug. By now it should feel nicely comfortable—if not a bit loose. You should also be noticing that your daily "fit" task is becoming much easier as your fitness level starts to build.

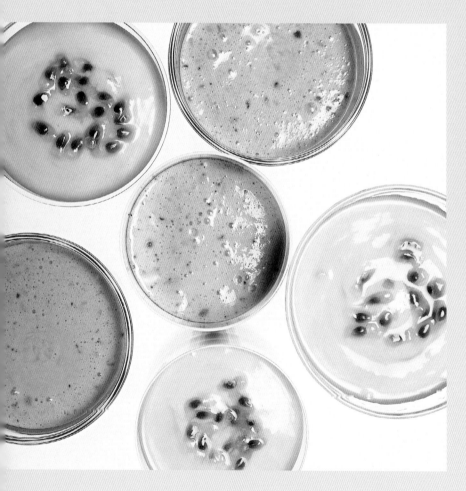

food
breakfast

breakfast smoothie
Made by blending together a handful of berries and ⅔ cup skim milk.

ALTERNATIVE
cranberry granola
(see page 72)
Serve with ¾ cup skim milk.

snack

2 oat biscuits topped with a very thin slice of low-fat cheese

lunch

falafels

4–5 falafels made according to the instructions on the package and served in a small whole-wheat pita with shredded lettuce, cucumber, and carrots and low-fat plain yogurt flavored with fresh mint.

ALTERNATIVE
tuna salad

2 oz canned tuna, drained, and served with a large helping of green salad, cherry tomatoes, 1 teaspoon low-calorie Italian salad dressing, and 4 seeded crisp breads.

dessert

slices of mango and cherries

snack

pear

dinner

turkey burgers

(see page 73)
Serve with multigrain rolls, tomato and red onion relish, and crisp salad leaves or roasted vegetables, such as bell peppers, mushrooms, eggplant, zucchini, and tomatoes.

ALTERNATIVE
vegetable stir-fry

Made from vegetables of your choice, served on 2 oz dried egg noodles. Add 1 teaspoon sweet chili sauce to taste.

dessert

instant whipped pudding

Make 1 portion from a package, using skim milk.

fit

Take some time to stretch. Lengthening the muscles not only helps release tension in the body, but also helps improve posture (and good posture makes you look actively 6½ pounds thinner).

A great morning and night stretch for your shoulders, legs, and upper body is to stand in a doorway with one arm resting on the door frame. Take a step forward and dip into as low a lunge as possible. Hold for 30–60 seconds, then repeat using the other arm.

feel good

Fluid retention is a common problem for many women—and adds extra weight on the scales and extra size to your waistline. To find out if you suffer from this, press your forefinger on your leg in three or four different places. If it stays white for more than a few seconds after you lift the finger away, you're carrying extra fluid.

Drinking 8 cups of water every day will help with this, but for an extra boost, add two cups of dandelion tea to your daily diet from now until the end of the plan. This is a natural diuretic, but unlike other diuretic drinks, it doesn't negatively interfere with your vitamin and mineral levels.

fact

GI eating really is suitable for the whole family—in fact, children who follow a low-GI diet tend to have less of a problem with obesity than other children. So your entire family can follow this plan, if you adjust the portion sizes to suit their appetites and activity levels.

cranberry granola

preparation: 10 minutes | **cooking:** 4–6 hours | **serves:** 4

1¾ cups rolled oats

⅓ cup dried cranberries

1 tablespoon sunflower oil

2 tablespoons honey

skim milk or low-fat plain yogurt, to serve

1 Place all the ingredients in a warm mixing bowl and stir until the oats are covered evenly with the oil and honey.

2 Turn out onto a nonstick baking plate, making sure that there are no lumps.

3 Place in the bottom of a warm oven, 200°F, for about 4–6 hours, stirring occasionally to prevent sticking or browning.

4 When crispy remove and allow to cool. Store in an airtight container. The mixture will keep fresh for several days if kept free of moisture.

5 Serve with skim milk or low-fat yogurt.

tip

Granola is very easy to make. You may also like to mix in a little ground cinnamon or ginger before baking.

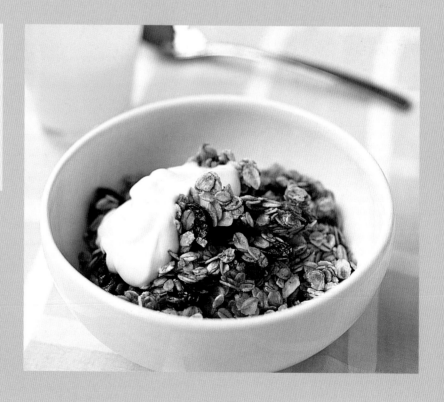

nutritional values per serving
Kcals **124 (523 kJ)**
Protein **2.8 g**
Carb **22.1 g**
Sodium **8 mg**
Fat **3.3 g**
Sat. fat **0.2 g**
GI **Low**

turkey burgers

preparation: 16 minutes plus chilling | **cooking:** 12–14 minutes | **serves:** 4

8 oz extra lean ground turkey

1 small onion, grated

2 small zucchini, grated

1 teaspoon soy sauce

1 egg

1 cup bread crumbs

¼ cup oatmeal

pepper

4 multigrain rolls, tomato and red onion relish, and crisp salad leaves or vegetables, to serve

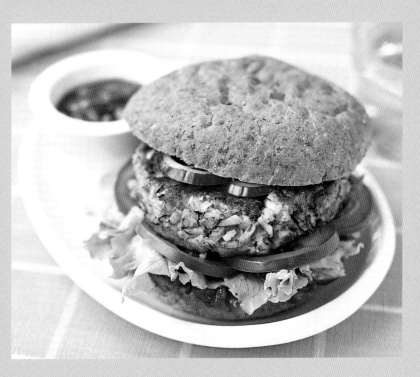

nutritional values per serving
Kcals **258 (1087 kJ)**
Protein **33.5 g**
Carb **20.7 g**
Sodium **214 mg**
Fat **5.1 g**
Sat. fat **1.1 g**
GI **Low**

1 Mix all the ingredients together in a bowl. Cover and leave in the refrigerator for 30 minutes. Divide the mixture into 4 and shape the burgers with your hands.

2 Preheat the broiler to medium. Line a broiler rack with foil and arrange the burgers on it. Cook for 6–7 minutes each side until thoroughly cooked.

3 Serve with multigrain rolls, tomato and red onion relish, and crisp salad leaves or a selection of roasted vegetables, such as bell peppers, mushrooms, zucchini, eggplant, and tomatoes.

day 12

Only three days to go now, so stay focused. Many people start to slip up towards the end of a diet plan, as their attention wanders and they start nibbling things from the refrigerator or using their eyes rather than their scales to determine portion sizes. Don't let this happen to you—remember, calories still count, even if you are eating low-GI foods.

food

breakfast

glass of red grapefruit juice
⅔ cup

bowl of bran cereal or low-sugar granola
3 tablespoons cereal with ¾ cup skim milk.

ALTERNATIVE
egg bagel
½ bagel topped with 1 egg, poached or scrambled with a little skim milk.

snack

2 oat biscuits spread with 1 teaspoon each of cottage cheese

lunch

pork and pineapple fajitas
(see page 77)

ALTERNATIVE
baked potato with tuna and corn
8 oz potato topped with 2 oz canned tuna and corn.

dessert

slice of melon

snack

packet of nuts, seeds, and raisins
3 tablespoons

dinner

oriental noodles
(see page 76)

ALTERNATIVE
soup followed by ham salad
7 oz can of tomato or vegetable soup 1 slice of lean ham (1 oz) with sliced tomatoes, cucumber, grated carrots, scallions, bell peppers, and lettuce. Serve with 4 large seeded rye crisp breads.

dessert

apricots with low-fat plain yogurt
Use either fresh apricots or canned apricots in their own juice.

fit

Try some "interval training." This fitness-boosting activity can be incorporated into whatever exercise you enjoy doing—be it cycling, walking, swimming, or jogging. To carry it out, every two to four minutes (depending on your fitness level) add a 30-second spurt, during which you work as hard as you can. Recover, then repeat. Do three or four of these spurts during your workout to strengthen your lungs and maximize the metabolic boost that the exercise gives you.

feel good

It's the end of the week and so, even with the potent fatigue-fighting powers of the GI plan, you could be feeling a little tired today. Revive yourself with a simple energizing acupressure technique. All you need to do is locate the little dips that appear around the hairline on the back of your neck, and about two finger widths on either side of your spine. Rest the fingers of each hand on the back of your head and use your thumbs to gently put pressure on this energizing point for 30 seconds.

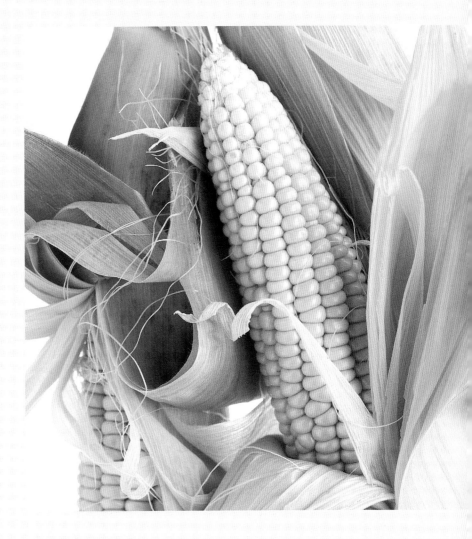

fact

Even if you don't keep up all your low-GI habits when the 14-day diet plan is over, simply adding a low-GI mid-morning snack to your day will help you feel more energized than normal.

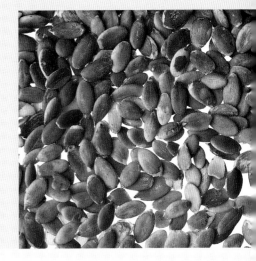

oriental noodles

preparation: 20 minutes | **cooking:** 15 minutes | **serves:** 4

½ cup light soy sauce

2 tablespoons dry rice wine vinegar

2 tablespoons plum sauce

1 lb lean pork tenderloin, cut into strips

8 oz dried medium egg noodles

4 small carrots

1 red bell pepper, cored and seeded

4 oz snow peas

6 oz baby corn

3 tablespoons sunflower oil

4 scallions, sliced

pepper

1 Mix together the soy sauce, vinegar, plum sauce, and some pepper in a shallow dish. Add the pork and coat well. Let stand for 30 minutes in a covered dish in the refrigerator.

2 Cook the noodles in boiling water for 5 minutes, then drain.

3 Cut the carrots into 2 inch batons. Slice the bell pepper into 2 inch strips. Blanch all the vegetables except the scallions for 2 minutes in boiling water and drain.

4 Heat the oil in a nonstick wok or pan. Stir-fry the pork until just browned. Add the blanched vegetables and cook quickly. Add the noodles and marinade. Stir-fry for 5 minutes.

5 Sprinkle with the scallions to serve.

tip

This is an easy recipe to make and it includes a good selection of vegetables. You can vary the vegetables and use zucchini, red kidney beans, frozen peas, and bean sprouts if you want. Nowadays you can buy pre-cooked noodles, which cuts down on the cooking time.

nutritional values per serving
Kcals **316 (1327 kJ)**
Protein **32.4 g**
Carb **15.1 g**
Sodium **591 mg**
Fat **13.9 g**
Sat. fat **2.8 g**
GI **Low**

pork and pineapple fajitas

preparation: 10 minutes | **cooking:** 10 minutes | **serves:** 4

½ **tablespoon olive oil**

1 **small onion, chopped**

7 **oz lean ground pork**

2 **garlic cloves, crushed**

1 **red bell pepper, cored, seeded and chopped**

4 **large mushrooms, sliced**

2 **canned pineapple rings, chopped**

2 **tablespoons pineapple juice**

1 **tablespoon tomato sauce**

1 **tablespoon soy sauce**

pinch of chili powder

2 **cups bean sprouts**

8 **tortilla wraps**

salad leaves, to serve

nutritional values per serving
Kcals **334 (1412 kJ)**
Protein **18.6 g**
Carb **56.7 g**
Sodium **419 g**
Fat **5.2 g**
Sat. fat **1.2 g**
GI **Low**

1 Heat the oil in a nonstick pan and fry the onion until soft.

2 Add the pork and the garlic to the pan and fry for 3–4 minutes until cooked.

3 Add all the other ingredients except for the bean sprouts and briskly fry for 3–4 minutes until softened.

4 Add the bean sprouts and, continually stirring, cook briskly for about 1–2 minutes.

5 Meanwhile, warm the tortilla wraps as directed on the package.

6 Spoon some of the pork mixture into the middle of each wrap and fold to contain the filling. Serve immediately, with salad leaves.

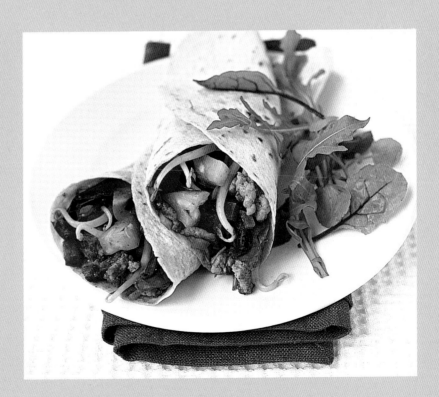

day 13

It's probably the weekend again, but this one shouldn't test your willpower too much. Partly because you've got only one more day on the plan to go, but also because now that you know how satisfied eating the GI way leaves you—and how energized you feel and how healthy you look while you follow its principles— there's no reason to cheat!

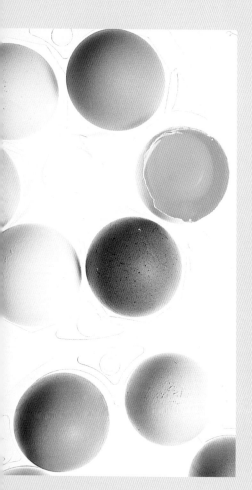

food

breakfast

glass of red grapefruit juice
⅔ cup

boiled egg and slice of granary toast

ALTERNATIVE
bowl of porridge
Made using 3 tablespoons rolled oats and ¾ cup water or skim milk. Top with a small banana.

snack

apple

lunch

chunky nut roast
(see page 80)

ALTERNATIVE
bought salad (under 300 calories) with broiled chicken and low-fat dressing

dessert

banana

snack

handful of plain peanuts and raisins
3 tablespoons

dinner

quick and easy risotto

Sweat sliced onions in a spray of olive oil in a large skillet and add a selection of vegetables, such as red bell peppers, mushrooms, and celery. Soften, then add ½ cup cooked basmati rice, 2 oz cooked chicken, peas and beans, 1 teaspoon tomato paste, oregano, and some water. Continue to cook until the water has evaporated and the vegetables are cooked.

ALTERNATIVE

pizza

Top a small 7 inch thin-crust pizza base with 2 tablespoons tomato pizza topping, ¼ cup low-fat grated cheese, and unlimited chopped onions. Serve with a large side salad of red bell pepper, broccoli florets, and 1 tablespoon corn.

dessert

whole-grain pancakes with cherries

(see page 81)

fit

Exercise doesn't need to involve shorts and trainers: gardening is a great calorie-burner and muscle-toner. If you've got a garden, head out there today and do some tidying—digging, weeding, and mowing the lawn (with a manual mower) are the best calorie-burners.

fact

Watch the salt content of foods such as rolled oats and other cereals—some are saltier than sea water. In an ideal world you should not eat more than ⅕ oz of salt a day: that's 2,400 mg of sodium. Check the labels of the foods that you choose carefully.

feel good

Spend a few minutes today reading the "What's On" section of your local paper and booking tickets for something next week. Anticipation has been shown to increase the levels of endorphins (the same mood-boosting hormones released when you exercise), which will help to keep you feeling good next week when you're off the plan—and, hopefully, will prevent you reaching for comfort foods to cheer yourself up.

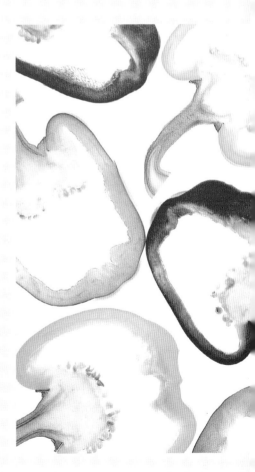

chunky nut roast

preparation: 15 minutes | **cooking:** 45 minutes | **serves:** 4

2 leeks, sliced

2 celery sticks, sliced

¾ cup chickpeas, cooked and roughly mashed

⅔ cup brown rice, cooked

½ cup mixed nuts, roughly chopped

2 teaspoons yeast extract

1 teaspoon chopped fresh mixed herbs

2 eggs, beaten

½ tablespoon low-fat spread

⅓ cup dried bread crumbs

salt and pepper

steamed broccoli and carrots, to serve

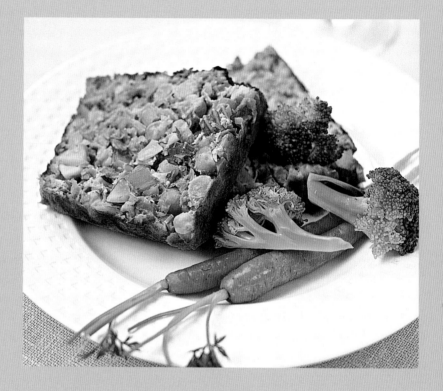

nutritional values per serving
Kcals **240 (1006 kJ)**
Protein **12.8 g**
Carb **21.2 g**
Sodium **576 mg**
Fat **12.2 g**
Sat. fat **2.3 g**
GI **Low**

1 Simmer the leeks and celery with a little water in a pan until soft. Allow to cool slightly.

2 Put the leeks and celery with the chickpeas, rice, nuts, yeast extract, herbs, and pepper into a bowl and mix. Then add the eggs and combine.

3 Line a 1 lb loaf pan with nonstick paper, grease well with low-fat spread and sprinkle with the bread crumbs. Spoon the mixture into the pan and level.

4 Bake uncovered in a preheated oven, 375°F, for 45 minutes until set.

5 Serve in slices with steamed broccoli and carrots.

whole-grain pancakes with cherries

preparation: 10 minutes plus standing | **cooking:** 16 minutes | **serves:** 4

¼ **cup whole-grain or whole-wheat flour**

¼ **cup all-purpose flour**

1 **egg, lightly beaten**

⅓ **cup skim milk**

1 **tablespoon vegetable oil**

fresh or canned cherries

low-fat plain yogurt and cinnamon, to serve

1 Sift the flours and add the egg and milk, stirring to make a batter the consistency of light cream. Add extra milk if the batter seems too thick, or extra flour if it seems too thin.

2 Allow to stand in a covered bowl in the refrigerator for 1 hour.

3 Heat the oil in a small nonstick skillet. Pour in a small amount of mixture and allow the mixture to run evenly over the base of the pan by lifting and turning it.

4 Cook on one side. Toss or lift and turn with a spatula to cook the other side. Repeat with the remaining mixture to make 8 thin pancakes. Keep the pancakes warm as they are made.

5 Stew cherries in a pan with a little water. If using cherries canned in syrup, rinse off the syrup first by washing the cherries in a strainer under a tap.

6 Top the pancakes with the stewed cherries and serve with plain yogurt and a sprinkling of cinnamon.

tip

This recipe can be varied by using other fruit, such as apples or pears. Or why not try a savory filling?

nutritional values per serving
Kcals **93 (369 kJ)**
Protein **3.8 g**
Carb **9.7 g**
Sodium **29 g**
Fat **4.6 g**
Sat. fat **0.8 g**
GI **Low**

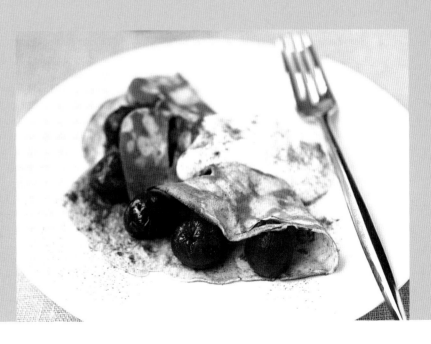

day 14

This is it, the last official day of your diet, and hopefully you've lost all the weight you want to. If you'd still like to lose a little more weight, you can either repeat the diet (using some of the recipe adaptation tips) or use the charts on pages 110–125 to help you devise your own low-GI menus. Try to keep to around 1,500 calories a day for women and 2,000 calories for men.

food

breakfast

glass of apple juice
⅔ cup

bowl of porridge
Made using 3 tablespoons rolled oats and ¾ cup water or skim milk.

ALTERNATIVE
poached egg and toast
Serve the egg with a slice of toasted sourdough, soy/linseed, or multigrain bread and broiled tomatoes.

snack

sunflower seeds
3 tablespoons

lunch

lemon and lime chicken with roasted vegetables
(see page 85)

ALTERNATIVE
roast vegetarian sausages and vegetables
2 roasted vegetarian sausages served with apple sauce, a mixture of 6 oz dry-roasted potatoes in their skins and sweet potatoes, carrots, peas, and Savoy cabbage.

dessert

red and green fruit salad
(see page 84)

snack

low-fat ice cream
¼ cup

dinner

mushroom omelet

Made with 2 eggs and served with a small whole-wheat pita bread and a large salad of leaves, sliced bell peppers, grated carrots, and a handful of mint tossed in lemon juice

ALTERNATIVE

pork stir-fry

Add a small (4 oz) broiled and sliced pork steak to a vegetable stir-fry made from a pack of stir-fry vegetables or a selection of snow peas, red and white onions, bean sprouts, noodles, oyster mushrooms, cherry tomatoes, and zucchini. Serve in a small whole-wheat pita bread.

dessert

2 pineapple rings and a handful of cherries

fact

Remember that by losing weight you've not only helped yourself look better, but you've also lowered your risk of developing problems such as heart disease, diabetes, and many cancers. Good for you!

fit

Why not make an appointment to go and see your local gym today? Most gyms will give you at least one trial session to see if you like it. At worst you'll get to do an hour of exercise—for example, trying a new class or testing out a strength-training regime such as weight training; at best you'll love it, join up and make exercise a part of your life from now on. Go on, give it a try.

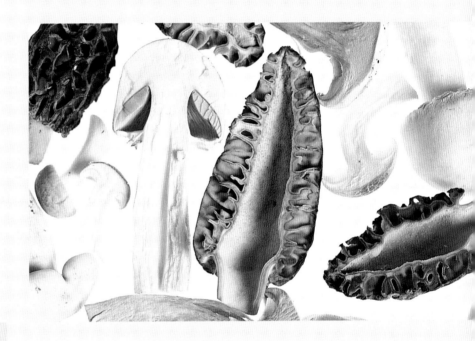

feel good

Take a look at the size of the portions on your plate today—and memorize them. Portion control isn't just the easiest way to keep off the weight that you've lost for longer; it's also, according to many experts, potentially the key to a longer life. Researchers studying the diets of the Okinawan people (thought to be the longest-lived race on Earth) have discovered that their small portions mean they eat about 1,500 calories a day (close to what you've been on for the last two weeks). If you stick to small portions it will prevent overtaxing your digestion, which can lead to fatigue, bloating, and belly ache.

red and green fruit salad

preparation: 10 minutes | **serves:** 4

4 kiwifruit

2 dessert apples, left unpeeled

1 pink grapefruit

handful of seedless green grapes, halved

4 tablespoons red berries

8 tablespoons low-sugar cranberry juice

low-fat plain yogurt, to serve

1 Slice the kiwifruit and apples and segment the grapefruit.

2 Mix in with the rest of the fruit and pour the cranberry juice over.

3 Serve with low-fat yogurt, allowing ¼ cup or about ½ pot per person.

nutritional values per serving
Kcals **74 (kJ 311)**
Protein **1.5 g**
Carb **16.6 g**
Sodium **6 mg**
Fat **0.5 g**
Sat. fat **0 g**
GI **Low**

tip

This easy recipe is also wonderful at breakfast time, and a very healthy way to start your day. You can alter the color combination by changing the fruits used.

lemon and lime chicken with roasted vegetables

preparation: 10 minutes | **cooking:** 1½ hours | **serves:** 4

3 lb chicken

3 lemons, 1 sliced

2 limes, 1 sliced

1 tablespoon vegetable oil

4 sweet potatoes, peeled and cut into chunks

4 zucchini, cut into chunks

2 onions, cut into chunks

1 large red bell pepper, cored, seeded, and cut into chunks

chicken gravy, to serve

1 Wash the chicken. Place 1 whole lemon inside. Slit the skin and insert the lemon and lime slices under the skin over the breast.

2 Place on a lightly greased baking sheet.

3 Cover with foil and roast in a preheated oven, 375°F, for 1⅓–1½ hours or until cooked. Remove the foil for the last 5 minutes and spoon the meat juices over. Check that the chicken is cooked —the juices should run clear

when a skewer is inserted through the thickest part of the leg and breast.

4 Cook the vegetables at the same time as the chicken. Put the oil in a baking dish. Add the vegetable chunks and squeeze the remaining lemon and lime over the top. Roast above the chicken for 1 hour.

5 Serve the chicken and vegetables with the gravy.

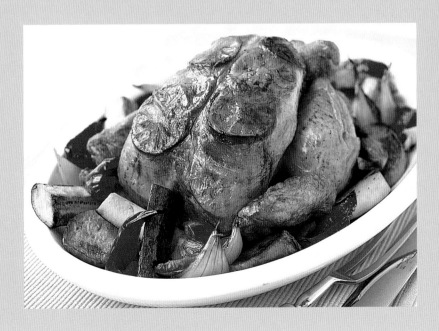

nutritional values per serving
Kcals **486 (kJ 2024)**
Protein **36.4 g**
Carb **25.6 g**
Sodium **150 g**
Fat **27.0 g**
Sat. fat **7.0 g**
GI **Low**

FIT

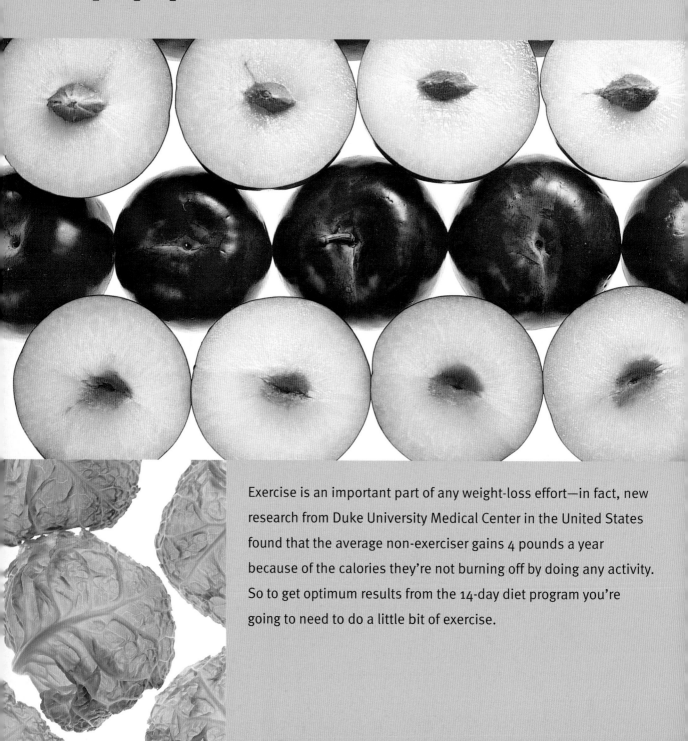

Exercise is an important part of any weight-loss effort—in fact, new research from Duke University Medical Center in the United States found that the average non-exerciser gains 4 pounds a year because of the calories they're not burning off by doing any activity. So to get optimum results from the 14-day diet program you're going to need to do a little bit of exercise.

If you've never exercised before, this might not be good news. But remember that exercise on a low-GI eating plan like this has been scientifically proven to feel easier than normal. All that slow-releasing glucose in your system is giving you the fuel you need to work out with less fatigue than usual; and burning more fat when you exercise after a low-GI meal means that any workout you do is more productive. Bearing these two facts in mind, here's exactly what you should be doing.

exercise beginner

On the next few pages you'll find a simple toning program that will help tighten and firm your muscles from head to toe. Each day you do a different workout to prevent your muscles getting tired. At the end of the week you start again with the first set of exercises—moving to the more advanced options if you feel up to it. Ideally, you should also do at least two of the daily "fit" tasks from the 14-day plan (see pages 30–85) each week; and/or choose one of the exercises suggested on pages 104–107 and carry it out for 30 minutes twice a week.

middle ground

If you already work out, you can power up your workout: either start with the more advanced options, repeating the same workout again during the second week, or replace it with your normal weights program at the gym. You can also do a "fit" task at least five times a week, and/or choose one of the exercises suggested on pages 104–107 and carry it out for 30–60 minutes three to five times a week.

super-fit

If you're already a regular exerciser, doing just one set of toning exercises a day might not be challenging enough. Either replace them with your normal weights program at the gym or, if you don't usually strength-train, carry out the suggested exercise plan each day, but combine two or three sets of exercises, using the advanced options. The next day choose two or three different sets to ensure that you're resting the muscles you worked yesterday. Repeat this approach for the next 14 days. In terms of aerobic work, you can complete a "fit" task each day, and/or choose one of the exercises suggested on pages 104–107 and carry it out for 30–60 minutes five times a week.

safe exercise is happy exercise

The exercises here can easily be done at home, with no special equipment except one simple dumb bell that you'll find at any sports store. However, do wear trainers, as they give your ankles some support. Each day offers an individual warm-up exercise that will help reduce the risk of injury, but ideally you should also walk or jog (depending on your fitness level) around the garden, up and down stairs, or even on the spot for five minutes before you start. Anyone who is very overweight or has health problems should consult their doctor or fitness professional before starting any exercise regime.

Exercising for life

Exercise is important for weight maintenance—without it the average person gains 4 pounds a year in extra weight. If you were a regular exerciser when you started this program, keep on doing what you did before you completed the 14-day plan.

Remember that your body gets used to the same workout if you do it too often, so think about incorporating one or two of the "fit" tasks into your workouts from now on. If, however, you were new to exercise when you started this plan, you may need a little more advice on how to progress.

The good news is that the hard bit is done, for you've started a workout program, so don't let things slip now. After your 14-day plan, keep up the daily toning for the next six weeks. At the end of that time, move up to the advanced options and keep doing them for six weeks. By then you'll have increased muscle tone and have sufficient flexibility to progress to trying out a toning exercise class or video that will challenge your

body and boost your results. In terms of the aerobic part of your workout (covered by the "fit" tasks in the diet plan), increasing the frequency and intensity of these will help keep your body challenged and will start to improve your fitness. Every three weeks add one more "fit" task to your week, until you're up to a task a day. Once you get to this point (or if you're there already), it's time to move on to more formal exercises, like those suggested on pages 90–103. Start with two or three 30–60-minute sessions a week, progressing to five sessions a week. But whatever you do, enjoy it—exercising positively affects every part of your body, so each session that you do boosts your health and helps you maintain your new slim shape.

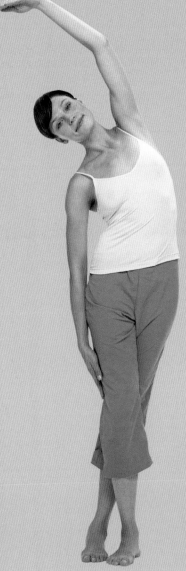

think yourself thin

While most people think losing weight is purely a physical matter, research is increasingly suggesting that putting your mind on your diet is just as important as eating the right foods—and vital when it comes to keeping off the weight. New research from the National Weight Control Registry in the US (which monitors the behavior of people who've successfully lost weight and kept it off) has discovered that people who think more dominantly with the logical, left half of their brain are more successful than creative, right-brain thinkers, leading them to believe that incorporating left-brain behavior into a weight-maintenance program is the key to success. So try the four tips here.

1 Plan more

Left-brainers are very precise and know what they're eating every day—and where it's coming from. Just going shopping with a list and never deviating from it will help.

2 Problem-solve

If you're continually finding that a particular situation is derailing your maintenance efforts (say you're always hungry after exercise and reach for the cookies, negating the calories you burned during your workout), think about what you could do to counteract this. Do you need a healthy snack before you work out, or should you ban all cookies from your home? Which solution works best for you?

3 Write things down

Left-brainers like to see things on paper. Once a month write down exactly what you've eaten, where you ate it, and how you felt beforehand. This can help you identify any extra calories or bad habits sneaking back into your plan.

4 Develop a routine

Establishing a set time of day to exercise or dedicating 20 minutes each morning to making your lunch will help you stay focused on your maintenance goals, and ensure that the weight you've lost stays gone—forever.

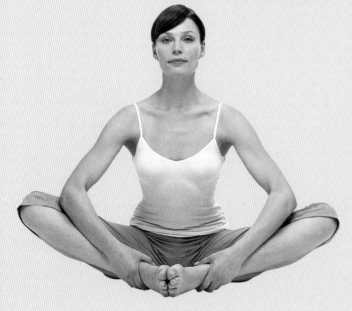

days 1 and 8

On days 1 and 8 of the program you're going to be focusing on two exercises that will strengthen your core muscles—those that lie around your abdominals. These are key to a healthy body but are also incredibly important as part of your fast fix: not only will strong, toned core muscles improve your posture, but a good posture will immediately make you look thinner.

warm-up exercise
the rotator

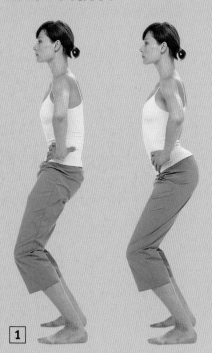

1

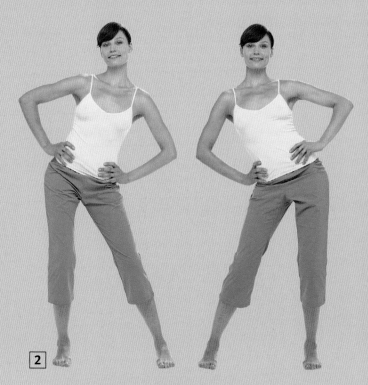

2

1 Stand with your feet hip-width apart and your hands on your hips. Push your hips from side to side, as if you are doing a dance. Now use your hands to tilt your pelvis forward and backward, tensing your stomach muscles to lift up your hips as you press your pelvis forward.

2 Move your feet further apart and bend your knees. Finally take your hips round in a full circle, first clockwise and then counterclockwise, using your stomach muscles to control the movement. Repeat the side-to-side, forward and backward movements and the revolutions twice.

toning exercise
the inch-up

Now that your mid-section is warmed up, you can perform the stomach-toning exercise really thoroughly.

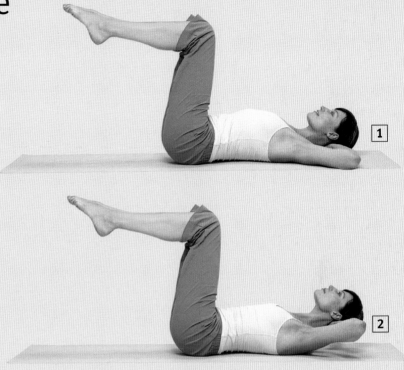

1 Lie on your back with your knees bent and your feet raised in the air. Place your hands behind your head, and try to relax your head into your hands.

2 Lift your head and shoulders off the floor to a count of one.

3 Now lift your head and shoulders higher off the floor and hold for a count of one; then inch them higher again and hold. Slowly release your head and shoulders back to the floor to a count of three. Repeat this exercise ten times in week one; in week two you should be trying to do more repetitions, or twice as many exercises.

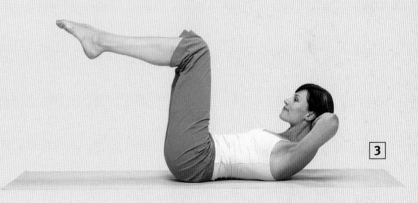

to finish

Spend five minutes jogging on the spot to boost your blood flow.

days 2 and 9

While strong core muscles support the body's posture, strong shoulder muscles are the key to standing in a way that creates the appearance of a svelte shape. Your shoulders should be dropped (not hunched upward) and your shoulder blades should be pulled down (not be rounded forward). These two exercises will help to strengthen the muscles that make this happen.

warm-up exercise
the swing-round

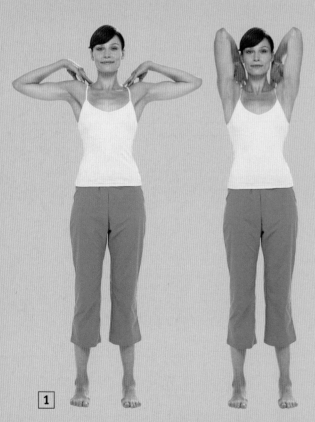

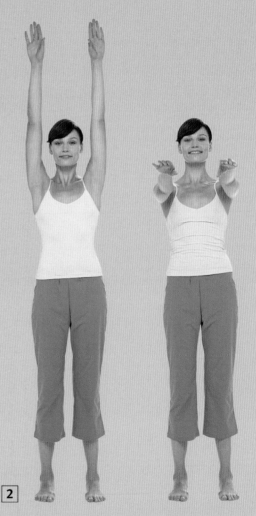

1 Put your hands on your shoulders. Lift your arms and draw circles with both elbows, so that you point them up to the ceiling, then around the back and down toward the floor. Keep your shoulders pressed down (squeeze your back muscles) as you do this.

2 Revolve your elbows twice, then extend your arms to complete two full circles with your arms outstretched.

toning exercise
the shoulder lift

Perform this exercise as many times as it takes to feel a real ache in your shoulders! The heavier the dumb-bell, the fewer repetitions you will need to do. When you have reached the "ache" point, rest for 20 seconds, then repeat the exercise the same number of times. In week two you should aim to increase the number of repetitions; this is also a good exercise of which to try at least one more complete set.

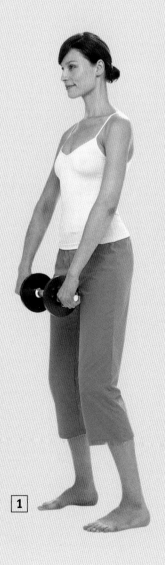

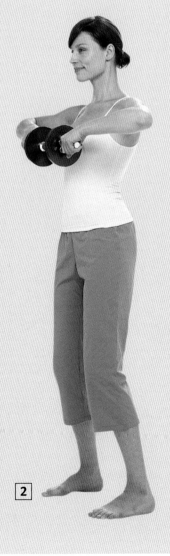

1 Grab hold of a 4–9 lb dumb-bell (you'll find these in any sports store), or you could use a large bottle of water as a substitute. Hold it with both hands in front of your body.

2 Now raise the dumb-bell to chest height, hold the position for two seconds and lower it again.

to finish

Spend five minutes hopping across the room, first on one leg and then on the other, to boost your lymphatic system.

days 3 and 10

On these days you start working on your leg muscles. Most of us already have some strength and tone in these, so they respond quickly to stimulation. However, both of the exercises here will also work the muscles at the back of the thighs and those in the buttocks, helping to firm up the main problem area for most women and to create stronger looking legs on most men.

warm-up exercise
the gentle squat

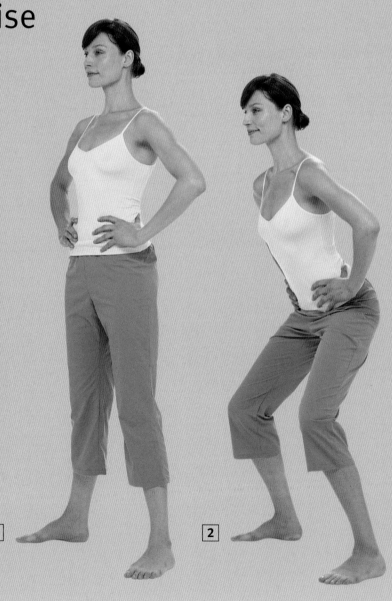

1 Stand with your legs wide apart and your hands on your hips. Now simply bend your knees—but not too far—pressing your knees out over your toes. Your buttocks should lower just behind your leg line.

2 Press your legs straight again, raising your body. Bend and straighten your legs several times, feeling the muscles in your thighs and trying to avoid any tension in your knees.

toning exercise
the held squat

Strengthening the muscles in your thighs and buttocks is a great way of keeping flab under control.

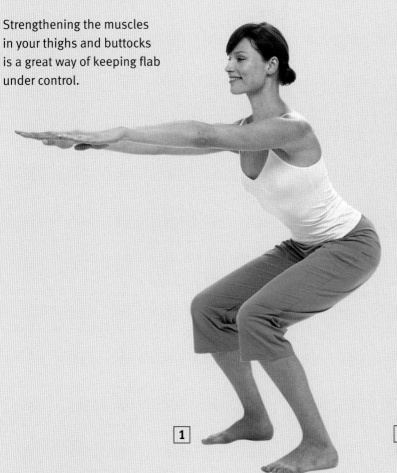

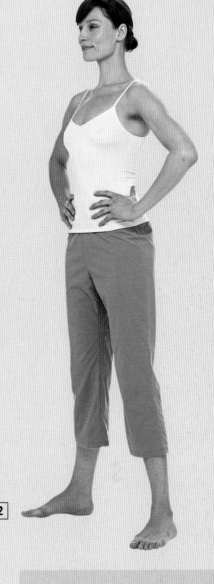

1 Turn your feet to a parallel position and place them hip-width apart. Stretch your arms out in front of you and squat down, bending your knees and lowering your buttocks behind you. Your legs should be bent, but not as far as 90 degrees.

2 Hold this lowered position, while inhaling for five breaths and feeling the muscles in your buttocks. Now press your legs straight, squeezing your buttocks to lift you up. Repeat ten times in week one; in week two you should aim to do more than this— or simply do two or three sets of ten repetitions.

to finish

Spend five minutes sprinting fast from one end of the garden (or park) to the other to boost your lung capacity.

days 4 and 11

Back to working on those core postural muscles again—this time focusing on the back muscles, particularly those that run along the spine. Many of us ignore these in favor of toning our tummies or thighs, but if the back muscles are weak, the whole body hangs out of alignment, which leads to pouchy stomachs and saggy gluteus muscles (and the buttocks they hold up).

warm-up exercise
the curve

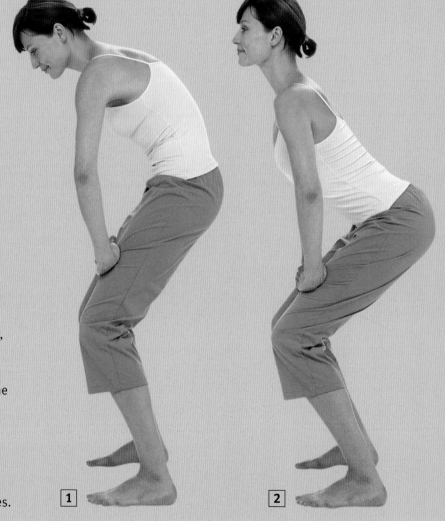

1 With your feet slightly apart and your hands on your thighs, bend your knees. Now curve your back, pulling in your stomach muscles as if someone has just punched you!

2 Flatten your back out again and press your buttocks out behind you. Repeat the curve-and-flatten technique five times.

toning exercise
the hyper-extension

This is an effective exercise for strengthening the muscles that run along the spine.

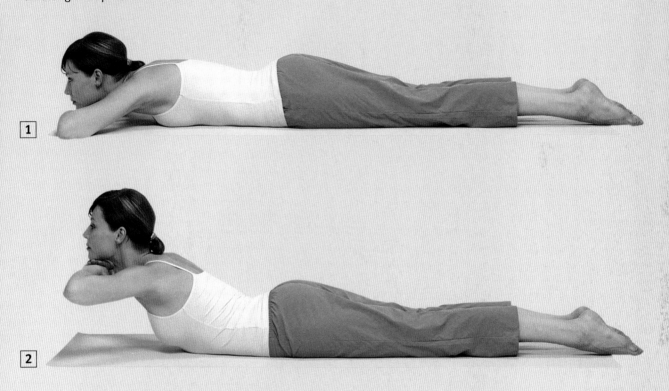

1 Lie on your front, with your arms resting on the floor in front of you and your head resting on your arms.

2 Now lift your head and hands up off the floor, and raise your shoulders and chest upward. Hold this lift for five breaths, before returning your upper body to the floor. Repeat the exercise ten times in week one; in week two either add five more repetitions, or relax after the first set and then repeat the exercise again ten times.

to finish

Spend five minutes jumping on the spot to boost your oxygen intake.

days 5 and 12

More leg work in this part of the program, but this time you're working the abductors and adductors—the muscles of the inner and outer thigh. Firming and toning these will create a smoother silhouette by reducing the look of those saddlebag bulges that can collect on the outside of the hips and thighs. These exercises also give an added boost to your buttock and thigh muscles.

warm-up exercise
the lunge walk

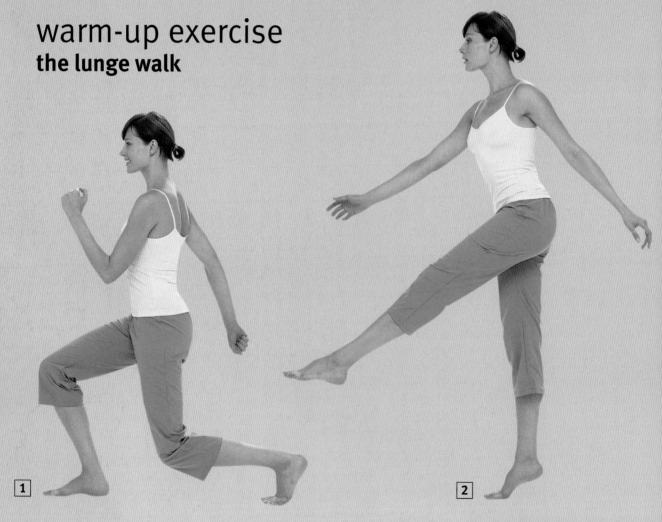

1 Step forward into a large step, bending low as you step.

2 Now push off vigorously into the next step forward. Do five large steps forward across the room and then five back again to warm up (and tone) your hip and buttock area.

toning exercise
the ball-buster

When you start to do this exercise you will feel your muscles being stretched. Be careful not to over-do it and strain yourself.

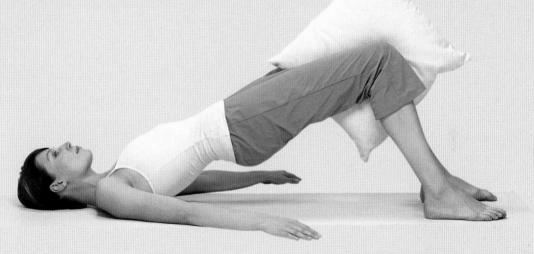

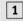

1 Lie on your back and place a ball between your knees (or a cushion, if don't have a ball), with your feet flat on the floor.

2 Squeeze your knees tightly against the object and lift your hips off the floor. Hold briefly, then lower yourself back to the floor. Repeat the lift-and-lower technique 12 times, then rest and repeat the set once more during the first week; and twice more during the second week, aiming to do 15 repetitions this week, if you can.

to finish

Spend five minutes dancing around the room to boost your feel-good factor by up to ten!

days 6 and 13

The backs of the arms are another area that is frequently ignored, but as your shoulders start to align into a better postural position, the backs of your arms can be pressed closer to your body and may actually start to look bigger than you would like them to. The good news is that a few simple exercises can have them tightened up and looking firmer in no time.

warm-up exercise
the side-shimmy

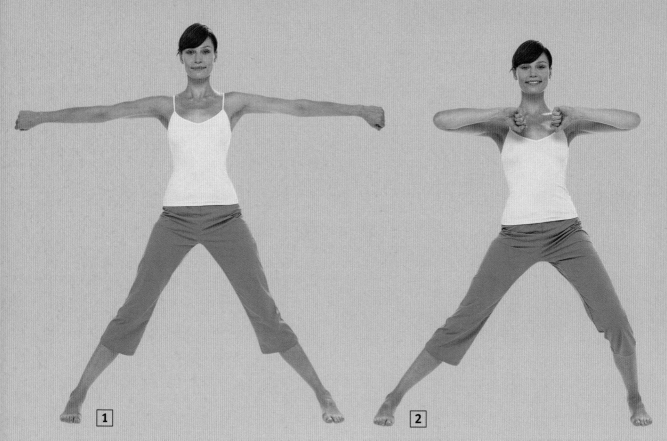

1 Stand with your legs wide apart and your arms extended out to each side, with palms facing back.

2 While bending your legs to one side and then the other, bend and straighten your arms, bringing your hands into your chest and out again. Do this 15 times, getting more vigorous each time.

toning exercise
the triceps trial

When you do this exercise, wedge your chair against a wall to make sure that it doesn't slip when you press against it.

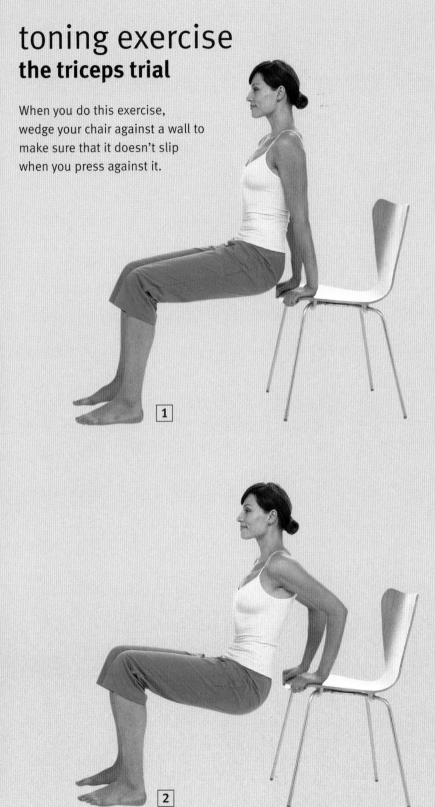

1 Sit on the edge of a chair or bench, with your hands on the edge of the seat and your feet flat on the floor. Now inch your buttocks off the chair, taking your weight onto your arms.

2 Lower your buttocks down toward the floor, then push with your arms to raise them up again. All the work here should be done by your arms, and not by your legs. Repeat up to ten times in week one; in week two take a rest after the first set, then repeat again, aiming to do eight to ten repetitions if you can.

to finish

Spend five minutes skipping (just like boxers do—you don't need a skipping rope) to boost your energy levels.

days 7 and 14

Finally it's time to work on the lower leg. Having and maintaining an erect posture hinges on having strength and correct positioning in the ankles, feet, and knees. So even though you might not worry about how they look in a bikini, it's important not to ignore these areas. These exercises are good for your circulation and will also help you create leaner, more shapely calf muscles.

warm-up exercise
tiptoe through the tulips

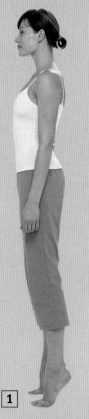

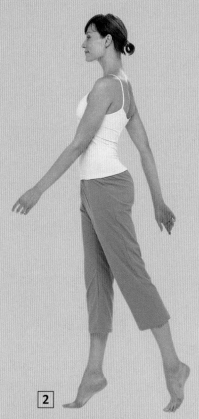

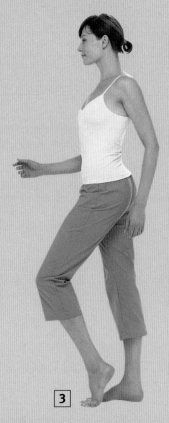

1 Stand on tiptoe and breathe normally to a count of five.

2 Walk on tiptoe from one side of the room to the other.

3 Now stand and press one heel to the floor and then the other. Raise and lower each heel in turn 10–15 times until your ankles and legs feel warm.

toning exercise
the jump

Don't look down as you do this series of jumps. Keep your eyes fixed straight ahead to help you with your balance.

1 Stand with your feet hip-width apart, then bend your knees and jump, swinging your arms as you do so. Aim to lift your feet right into the air and stretch them underneath you. Try to land on the balls of your feet and let the rest of your feet roll onto the floor as you land, bending your knees to absorb the shock.

2 Now repeat the exercise, but don't push yourself right off the floor—your toes should stay in contact with it. Repeat both exercises eight times, then rest and repeat a further three times in week one to shape the calves. In week two do 10–15 raises, again repeating them three times.

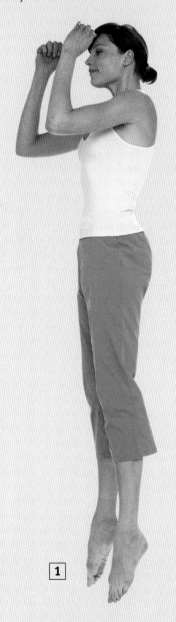

1

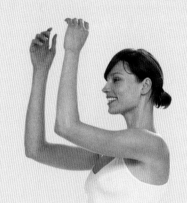
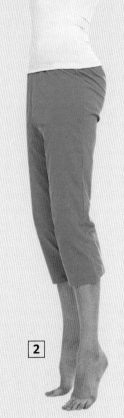

2

to finish

Spend five minutes lying flat on the floor with your feet raised on a bed or bench and your head lower than your feet to boost the blood flow to your brain and help reduce fluid retention in your lower legs.

Calories burned

Remember, the bigger the gap between the number of calories you eat each day and those you burn, the more weight you lose on a slimming regime. Every time you move you burn calories, but obviously some activities are better at this than others.

This chart explains how many calories a 150 pound woman will burn doing some common daily tasks or fitness activities; men and women who weigh more than this will burn more calories—to calculate exactly how many, divide the number of calories listed by 150, and then multiply it by your weight in pounds. Depending on your fitness level, you could replace any of your daily "fit" tasks with 30–60 minutes of any of these activities.

ACTIVITY	CALORIES/KCAL PER 15 MINUTES	ACTIVITY	CALORIES/KCAL PER 15 MINUTES	ACTIVITY	CALORIES/KCAL PER 15 MINUTES
Aerobics	95	Cycling (outside—moderate)	158	Jogging	125
Aikido (intense)	158	Dancing (general)	70	Judo	158
Aqua aerobics	77	Darts	39	Kayaking (moderate)	79
Archery	55	Digging	100	Kick-boxing	158
Ashtanga yoga	100	Downhill skiing	79	Lawn mowing (push mower)	87
Badminton	71	Driving	27	Line-dancing	70
Basketball	95	Dusting	40	Mopping the floor	45
Bathing the dog	66	Fishing	63	Mountain biking	135
Billiards	39	Football	100	Moving furniture	90
Bowling	47	Gardening	80	Netball	95
Boxing	142	Golf (with cart)	45	Painting (interior)	71
Canoeing	120	Golf (without cart)	60	Papering walls	48
Carpentry	55	Gymnastics	63	Pilates (light)	50
Carrying shopping	63	Hatha yoga	40	Pilates (moderate)	75
Cleaning the house	39	Hiking	95	Pilates (intense)	100
Climbing stairs	150	Hockey	100	Playing tag	80
Cooking	27	Ice hockey	130	Power-walking	103
Cricket	79	Ice skating (moderate)	75	Pushing a baby buggy	39
Cross-country skiing	125	Indoor climbing	175	Raking leaves	72
Cycling (on an exercise bike)	79	Irish step-dancing	87	Resistance bands	75

ACTIVITY	CALORIES/KCAL PER 15 MINUTES	ACTIVITY	CALORIES/KCAL PER 15 MINUTES	ACTIVITY	CALORIES/KCAL PER 15 MINUTES
Rock-climbing	175	Squash (intense)	212	Toning tables	55
Rounders	79	Stairmaster machine	145	Treadmill running	140
Rowing (machine)	137	Standing	25	Treadmill running (on 5% incline)	160
Rowing (outside)	175	Step aerobics	140	Vacuuming	45
Rugby	158	Stretching	40	Volleyball	127
Sailing	47	Stripping wallpaper	48	Walking (normal pace)	55
Scrubbing the floor	87	Sweeping the floor	65	Walking (brisk)	63
Shopping	45	Sweeping the path	70	Washing dishes	45
Shoveling snow	106	Swimming (breaststroke)	95	Washing the car	64
Sit-ups	63	Swimming (butterfly)	175	Weight training	54
Skipping	175	Swimming (front crawl)	125	Window cleaning	45
Snorkeling	79	Tai chi	63	Windsurfing	50
Spinning class	160	Tennis (doubles)	95		
Sprinting	214	Tennis (singles)	160		

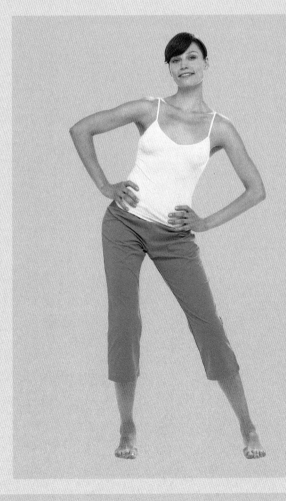

how hard is too hard?

The harder you do any activity, the more calories you'll burn. However, if you work out too hard for your fitness level, you'll get too tired to gain the maximum benefit. And you burn a higher proportion of fat if you work out at about 70 percent of your maximum ability. So whenever you do any exercise on this plan (or generally in life) you should aim to be working at a level that feels like roughly six or seven out of ten. Or use the "talk test" discussed briefly on page 55: you should be working hard enough to be able to speak in sentences, but should feel the need to take a break between them.

Fun activities

Still not convinced that working out is right for you? Then make your daily "fit" task something fun. None of the activities below feels like exercise, but they all help you tone and burn calories. Go on—give one or two of them a try over the next 14 days.

archery
Burning 220 calories an hour, it's easy to see why archery creates firm arm muscles and helps sculpt a strong upper back. Other fitness boosts include dramatically improved posture and tightened tummy muscles. It won't help your aerobic fitness, though, so don't make it your only workout.

belly-dancing
Not only does it burn around 381 calories an hour, but it also helps tone the muscles of the stomach, waist, hips, and thighs. Videos teaching the technique are available; or look in your local newspaper or at your local sports center to see if classes are offered.

boogie-boarding
A great sport for anyone who lives near a beach. All you need is a small, light board; you then run into the waves and lie on the board to surf your way back in.

Running against the resistance of the water helps tone your legs, while staying on the board requires tight, toned tummy muscles.

dancing video games
These are played on a home games system and burn a staggering 600 calories an hour, if you get good at it. You stand on a mat with sensors and get your instructions onscreen as to what steps to do—and are scored for accuracy. Your local computer games store can tell you more about what you need to get started.

flamenco
Or salsa, or ballroom ... Dance classes are a gentle way for people who don't normally exercise to start improving their fitness, without the pressure of visiting a gym. They burn a minimum of 200 calories an hour, and you'll also slim your legs and improve your posture.

frisbee
This sport is even better for your body shape if you're bad at it—the more you run after the frisbee and reach over to pick it up, the more calories you burn (on average around 200 an hour). Jumping to catch the disk also causes rapid toning of buttocks and thighs.

horseriding
Burning around 280 calories an hour, riding firms up the thighs, buttocks, and stomach. But the calorie-burning doesn't stop when you dismount; grooming a horse will burn around 200 calories in half an hour. If you've never ridden before, take a few lessons—if you're a natural, you'll be trotting in a month or less.

hula-hooping
If you want to flatten your tummy fast, this is the exercise for you. You have to hold in your

stomach muscles to keep the hoop rotating—and you'll burn about 300 calories an hour while having fun. For extra benefits, think about using a weighted hoop (available from sports stores) to intensify your workout.

in-line skating

This gives your heart and lungs a similar level of workout to running, but you don't feel as if you're working anything like as hard, because the wind helps keep you cool and there's no impact on your joints to cause pain. An hour's skate will burn 480 calories.

kite-flying

A great activity to do with children, stationary kite-flying will burn only 100 calories an hour. Get yourself a sports kite in a high wind, however, and that could increase to 250 calories as you twist and turn to catch the wind—and run (or at least walk briskly) to pick up your kite when it falls.

pedal-boating

You'll find pedal boats in local parks and, while they may look simple, they give you the same workout as sitting on a type of exercise bike called a recumbent and pedaling it on medium resistance. As a result you'll burn about 300 calories in an hour—and work your legs and buttock muscles.

playgrounding

Also known as "playing with your children," this will have you clambering on the climbing frame, spinning the roundabout, pushing them on the swings, and running round the playground as if you were six again. Burning around 350 calories an hour, this is another great way to involve your children in your fitness efforts.

snowboarding

You don't need to live near a mountain to do this—many indoor ski slopes offer lessons, too. It's said to be easier to learn than skiing (as both legs are on the same piece of equipment) and all you need to succeed is good balance. An hour's session will burn around 350 calories.

table tennis

A fast game of table tennis can be such a good workout that it's now being rebranded "Killer Spin." For most of us, though, it's just a nice way to have fun with the kids. The more you move around the table and reach for shots, the greater its fitness effects; you could expect to burn 250 calories in an hour-long tournament.

trampolining

Toning buttocks and thighs and speeding up the lymph system (which helps flush fluid and toxins out of the body), trampolining is one of those exercises where you don't realize how hard you're working because you're laughing so much. But you are working hard: manage 30 minutes and you'll burn 150–200 calories.

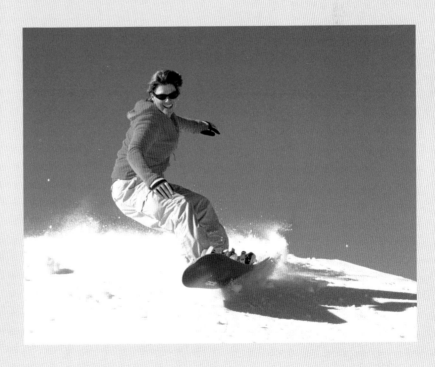

FOREVER

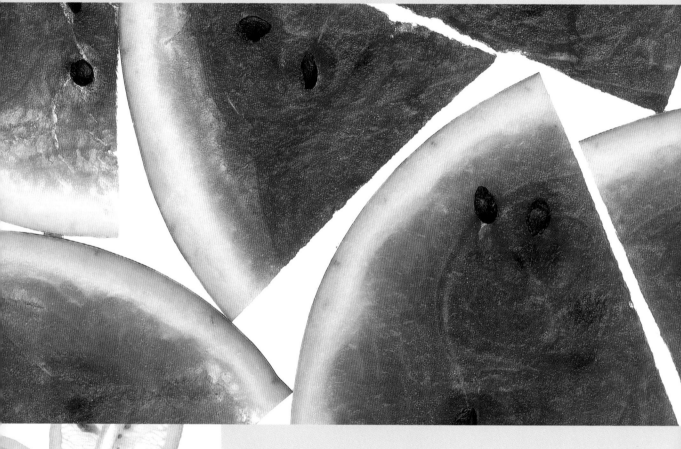

So that's it: your 14-day plan is finished, and hopefully you're thrilled with the results. What now? Well, if you've got more weight to lose, turn back to pages 24–25 for tips on how to adapt the diet for longer term weight loss or use the charts on the following pages to create your own eating plan. If you've achieved the weight loss you wanted, congratulations—you've taken the first step to that slimmer new you. So what exactly should you eat from now on to keep it that way?

low-GI for life

Many fast-fix weight-loss plans simply don't teach you what to eat once the weight has come off. This plan isn't like that. Because all the food groups are included, you don't feel as if you're missing out on things, and the inclusion of desserts and "high-fat" foods like chocolate, nuts, and seeds helps you appreciate that you can have higher calorie treats and still stay slim. So eating the low-GI way for life is relatively easy.

To determine exactly what you should eat, you can use two maintenance tools. The box on this page tells you how to adapt the GI pyramid from pages 20–21 to maintain your weight, and the charts on the following pages will help you mix and match your own eating choices to tailor that pyramid to your likes and dislikes. A few final facts will help you incorporate higher GI foods into your eating plan without adversely affecting your blood-sugar levels.

1 Try not to have more than one high-GI food a day. Two weeks of low-GI eating will have stabilized your blood-sugar levels and reduced the amount of insulin in your system. However, if you start overloading your system with high-GI foods, the situation will reverse, your energy levels will fall, and you could find yourself overeating and the weight going back on.

2 If you do eat a high-GI food, combining it with a low-GI food will reduce the speed at which the high-GI one converts to sugar. So if you treat yourself to some crusty French bread or mashed potato, eat it with a little fat, protein, or a selection of vegetables to help lower the GI.

3 Keep portions of all carbohydrates sensible. The more of a particular food you eat, the more glucose is produced, so to avoid overloading your system keep portion sizes to those suggested on pages 22–23.

the GI maintenance pyramid

The GI pyramid (see page 21) indicates the overall proportions of the different food groups that you should eat each day when you're trying to diet. However, it's a bit restrictive once you've lost the weight, so you can amend it as follows:

• The high-GI, low-nutrient foods in the top section can be enjoyed 1–2 times a week.

• The high-GI, higher-nutrient foods in the second layer can be eaten once a day.

• The next sections (nuts and seeds, dairy and protein foods) should remain the same.

• You can now increase the carbohydrates you eat and incorporate up to two portions of medium-GI foods, such as couscous or brown rice. Women should stick to 6–8 servings, while men can eat up to 11 (remember that any high-GI carbs should be included in this total).

• Fruit and vegetables should stay the same, aiming for at least 5 portions a day—ideally in a 3:2, vegetable: fruit ratio.

GI chart

This chart shows the energy content of foods per 3½ oz as kcal (kilocalories) and kJ (kilojoules).The GI value of foods is also shown, together with whether the food in question is high, medium, or low in GI terms. It should be noted that the GI values can vary between varieties of fruits and vegetables and different manufacturers, and according to the way in which items are cooked. The value for both cooked and raw items has been given if they are commonly served as such. Remember that where possible it is better to steam vegetables as this helps to retain the vitamin content. The values given here remain the same for boiling and steaming.

	KCAL	KJ	GI VALUE		KCAL	KJ	GI VALUE
A				**B**			
Alfalfa	24	100	1 low	**Bacon,** broiled	337	1400	0 low
Anchovies, canned in oil	191	798	0 low	**Bacon,** Canadian, broiled	287	1194	0 low
Angler fish, broiled	96	407	0 low	**Bacon,** Canadian, reduced salt, broiled	282	1172	0 low
Apple	47	199	38 low	**Bagel,** white	273	1161	72 high
Apple juice, unsweetened	38	164	40 low	**Baked beans**	84	355	48 low
Apricots, canned in juice	34	147	64 med	**Baked beans,** reduced sugar and salt	73	311	48 low
Apricots, dried	188	802	30 low				
Apricots, fresh	31	134	57 med	**Baked potato**	136	581	85 high
Artichoke, boiled	18	77	1 low	**Baking powder**	157	693	0 low
Artichoke, canned	28	119	1 low	**Banana**	95	403	52 low
Asparagus, steamed	26	110	1 low	**Barley, pearl,** boiled	120	510	25 low
Avocado	190	784	1 low	**Basmati rice,** boiled	138	587	58 med
				Bean sprouts, raw	31	131	1 low

	KCAL	KJ	GI VALUE		KCAL	KJ	GI VALUE
Bean sprouts, stir-fried	72	298	1 low	**Beef, corned**, canned	205	860	0 low
				Beef, grillsteaks, broiled	305	1268	0 low
BEANS AND LEGUMES				**Beef,** hamburgers 99% meat, broiled	326	1353	0 low
Baked beans	84	355	48 low	**Beef,** round steak stewed	185	777	0 low
Baked beans, reduced sugar and salt	73	311	48 low	**Beef,** sirloin steak, lean fried	183	770	0 low
Black-eyed beans, soaked and boiled	116	494	42 low	**Beef,** sirloin steak, lean broiled	177	745	0 low
Buckwheat, boiled	364	1522	54 low	**Beet,** boiled	46	195	80 high
Chickpeas, canned	115	487	42 low	**Black-eyed beans,** soaked and boiled	116	494	42 low
Chickpeas, soaked and boiled	121	512	28 low	**Bouillon cube,** chicken	237	990	1 low
Fava beans, steamed	48	204	61 med	**Bouillon cube,** vegetable	253	1055	1 low
Green beans, raw	24	99	1 low	**Bran cereal,** flakes	330	1406	74 high
Green beans, steamed	25	108	1 low	**Bran cereal,** noodle-shaped	270	1144	34 low
Kidney beans, canned	100	424	36 low				
Kidney beans, soaked and boiled	100	424	28 low	**BREADS, CAKES, AND PASTRY**			
Lentils, green, canned	64	273	48 low	**Bagel,** white	273	1161	72 high
Lentils, green, soaked and boiled	105	446	30 low	**Chocolate cake**	456	1908	38 low
Lentils, red, soaked and boiled	100	424	26 low	**Croissant**	373	1563	67 med
Lima beans, canned	77	327	36 low	**Crumpet**	177	753	69 med
Lima beans, soaked and boiled	103	437	31 low	**Fruit bread**	295	1256	47 low
Soy beans, boiled	141	590	20 low	**Fruit cake**	371	1561	54 low
Split peas, soaked and boiled	126	538	32 low	**Multigrain bread**	237	1005	61 med
				Pancakes	302	1265	67 med
				Pastry	451	1884	59 med

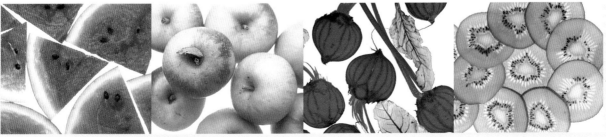

	KCAL	KJ	GI VALUE		KCAL	KJ	GI VALUE
Pita bread, white	255	1084	57 med	**Butter**	744	3059	0 low
Pretzels	381	1596	83 high				
Rye bread, no grains	219	932	51 low	**C**			
Rye/pumpernickel bread, with grains	219	932	41 low	**Cabbage,** raw	26	109	1 low
				Cabbage, steamed	16	67	1 low
Scones, plain	364	1530	92 high	**Camembert cheese**	290	1205	0 low
Soy/linseed bread	252	1070	41 low	**Carrots,** raw	35	146	49 low
Sponge cake	467	1951	46 low	**Carrots,** steamed	24	100	31 low
Waffles	334	1401	76 high	**Cauliflower,** boiled	28	117	1 low
White bread	235	1002	70 high	**Cauliflower,** raw	34	142	1 low
Whole-wheat bread	217	922	77 high	**Celery,** raw	7	30	0 low
				Celery, steamed	8	34	0 low

BREAKFAST CEREALS

	KCAL	KJ	GI VALUE
Bran cereal, flakes	330	1406	74 high
Bran cereal, noodle-shaped	270	1144	34 low
Chocolate rice cereal	383	1632	77 high
Cornflakes	376	1601	77 high
Muesli, Swiss	363	1540	56 med
Rice cereal, plain	382	1628	82 high
Rolled oats, dried	401	1698	42 low
Weetabix	352	1498	69 med
Wheat cereal	89	376	0 low

	KCAL	KJ	GI VALUE
Cheddar cheese	416	1725	0 low
Cheddar cheese, low-fat	273	1141	0 low

CHEESES

	KCAL	KJ	GI VALUE
Camembert	290	1205	0 low
Cheddar	416	1725	0 low
Cheddar, low-fat	273	1141	0 low
Cottage cheese	101	423	0 low
Cottage cheese, low-fat	79	334	0 low
Cream cheese	439	1807	0 low
Edam	341	1416	0 low
Edam, low-fat	229	957	0 low
Feta	250	1037	0 low
Mozzarella	257	1067	0 low
Parmesan	415	1729	0 low

	KCAL	KJ	GI VALUE
Broccoli, green, boiled	24	100	1 low
Broccoli, green, raw	33	138	1 low
Brussels sprouts, steamed	35	153	1 low
Buckwheat, boiled	364	1522	54 low

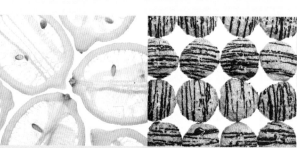
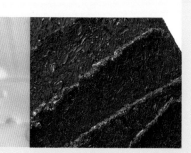

	KCAL	KJ	GI VALUE		KCAL	KJ	GI VALUE
Stilton	410	1698	0 low	Condensed milk	333	1406	61 med
Cherries	48	203	22 low	**COOKIES AND CRACKERS**			
Chicken, breast, no skin broiled	148	626	0 low	Graham crackers	465	1956	59 med
Chicken, drumsticks roasted	185	775	0 low	Oatcakes	412	1737	54 low
				Rice cakes, white	374	1591	82 high
Chicken, meat and skin roasted	216	912	0 low	Shortbread	509	2133	64 med
Chicken, strips, stir-fried	161	677	0 low	Corn, boiled	66	280	48 low
Chickpeas, canned	115	487	42 low	Corn, canned	23	96	46 low
Chickpeas, soaked and boiled	121	512	28 low	Corn chips	459	1927	42 low
				Corn kernels, boiled	111	470	48 low
Chips, potato	530	2215	57 med	Corned beef, canned	205	860	0 low
Chocolate, dark	510	2137	41 low	Cornflakes	376	1601	77 high
Chocolate, milk	520	2177	42 low	Cottage cheese	101	423	0 low
Chocolate cake	456	1908	38 low	Cottage cheese, low-fat	79	334	0 low
Chocolate mousse	149	627	37 low	Couscous, cooked	227	950	65 med
Chocolate mousse, low-fat	123	518	31 low	Crab, canned in brine	77	326	0 low
				Crab meat, boiled	128	535	0 low
Chocolate rice cereal	383	1632	77 high	Cranberry juice	61	259	52 low
Cockles, boiled	53	226	0 low	Cream cheese	439	1807	0 low
Coconut oil	899	3696	0 low	Croissant	373	1563	67 med
Cod fillet, baked	96	408	0 low	Crumpet	177	753	69 med
Coffee, black	0	0	0 low	Cucumber	10	40	1 low
Cola	41	174	53 low	Custard powder, made with skim milk	95	404	35 low
Cola, diet	0	0	0 low				
Collard greens, raw	33	136	1 low	Custard powder, made with whole milk	118	492	35 low
Collard greens, steamed	20	82	1 low				

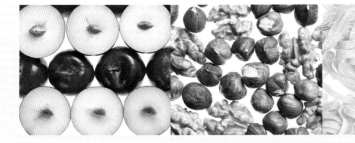
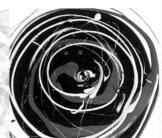

D

DAIRY PRODUCTS

	KCAL	KJ	GI VALUE
Condensed milk	333	1406	61 med
Custard powder, made with skim milk	95	404	35 low
Custard powder, made with whole milk	118	492	35 low
Ice cream, full-fat	177	741	61 med
Ice cream, low-fat	119	499	50 low
Skim milk	32	136	32 low
Soy milk	32	132	36 low
Soy yogurt	72	305	50 low
Whole milk	66	274	31 low
Yogurt, low-fat	56	237	33 low
Yogurt, low-fat, fruit	78	331	31 low
Yogurt, virtually fat-free, diet	54	230	20 low
Dates, dried	270	1151	103 high
Diet cola	0	0	0 low

DRINKS

	KCAL	KJ	GI VALUE
Apple juice, unsweetened	38	164	40 low
Coffee, black, no sugar	0	0	0 low
Cola	41	174	53 low
Cola, diet	0	0	0 low
Cranberry juice	61	259	52 low

	KCAL	KJ	GI VALUE
Grapefruit juice, unsweetened	33	140	48 low
Orange juice, unsweetened	36	153	53 low
Pineapple juice, unsweetened	41	177	46 low
Tea, black	0	0	0 low
Tea, herbal	0	0	0 low
Tomato juice, no added sugar	14	62	38 low
Water	0	0	0 low
Duck, crispy Chinese	331	1375	0 low
Duck, meat and skin roasted	388	1603	0 low
Duck, meat only, roasted	195	815	0 low

E

	KCAL	KJ	GI VALUE
Edam cheese	341	1416	0 low
Edam cheese, low-fat	229	957	0 low
Eels, jellied	98	406	0 low
Egg noodles, boiled	62	264	46 low
Eggplant, fried	302	1246	1 low
Eggs	151	627	0 low
Eggs, boiled	151	627	0 low
Eggs, fried	179	745	0 low
Eggs, omelet, cheese	271	1121	0 low
Eggs, omelet, plain	195	808	0 low
Eggs, poached	147	612	0 low

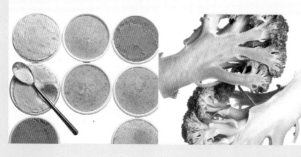
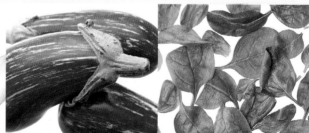

	KCAL	KJ	GI VALUE		KCAL	KJ	GI VALUE
Eggs, scrambled	257	1062	0 low	**Salmon,** canned in brine	153	644	0 low
Egg white	6	153	0 low	**Salmon,** canned in oil	153	644	0 low
				Salmon, smoked	142	598	0 low
F				**Salmon,** steamed	194	812	0 low
Fava beans, steamed	48	204	61 med	**Sardines,** canned in oil	220	918	0 low
Fennel, boiled	11	47	1 low	**Sardines,** fresh, broiled	195	815	0 low
Fennel, raw	12	50	1 low	**Scallops,** steamed	118	501	0 low
Feta cheese	250	1037	0 low	**Shrimp,** canned in brine	94	398	0 low
Figs, dried	227	967	61 med	**Shrimp,** frozen	73	310	0 low
				Shrimp, peeled and boiled	99	418	0 low
FISH AND SHELLFISH							
Anchovies, canned in oil	191	798	0 low	**Sole fillet,** steamed	91	384	0 low
Angler fish, broiled	96	407	0 low	**Swordfish,** broiled	139	583	0 low
Cockles, boiled	53	226	0 low	**Trout fillet,** broiled	135	565	0 low
Cod fillet, poached	94	396	0 low	**Tuna,** canned in brine	99	422	0 low
Crab, canned in brine	77	326	0 low	**Tuna,** canned in oil	189	794	0 low
Crab meat, boiled	128	535	0 low				
Flounder, broiled	96	404	0 low	**Flounder,** broiled	96	404	0 low
Haddock, steamed	89	378	0 low	**Frankfurter,** ready-cooked	287	1189	0 low
Halibut, broiled	121	513	0 low				
Kippers, broiled	161	667	0 low	**FRUIT**			
Lobster, boiled	103	435	0 low	**Apple**	47	199	38 low
Mackerel, fresh, fried	272	1130	0 low	**Apple juice,** unsweetened	38	164	40 low
Mussels, boiled, no shells	28	119	0 low	**Apricots,** canned in juice	34	147	64 med
Mussels, boiled, with shells	104	440	0 low	**Apricots,** dried	188	802	30 low
				Apricots, fresh	31	134	57 med
Oysters, raw	65	275	0 low	**Avocado**	190	784	1 low

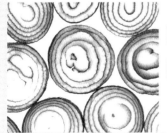
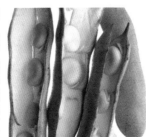
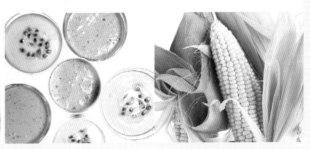

	KCAL	KJ	GI VALUE
Banana	95	403	52 low
Cherries	48	203	22 low
Figs, dried	227	967	61 med
Fruit cocktail, canned in syrup	57	244	55 low
Golden raisins	275	1171	56 med
Grapefruit	30	126	25 low
Grapefruit juice, unsweetened	33	140	48 low
Grapes, red	60	257	53 low
Grapes, white	60	257	53 low
Kiwifruit	49	207	53 low
Mango	57	245	51 low
Orange	37	158	42 low
Orange juice, unsweetened	36	153	53 low
Papaya	36	153	56 med
Peaches, canned in juice	39	165	40 low
Pears, canned in juice	33	141	45 low
Pineapple, canned in juice	47	200	46 low
Pineapple, fresh	41	176	66 med
Pineapple juice, unsweetened	41	177	46 low
Plums	34	145	34 low
Prunes	141	601	29 low
Raisins	272	1159	64 med

	KCAL	KJ	GI VALUE
Rhubarb, stewed	7	30	0 low
Tomato juice, no added sugar	14	62	38 low
Watermelon, no skin	31	133	72 high
Fruit bread	295	1256	47 low
Fruit cake	371	1561	54 low
Fruit cocktail, canned in syrup	57	244	55 low

G

	KCAL	KJ	GI VALUE
Gelatin	338	1435	0 low
Ghee	895	3693	0 low
Golden raisins	275	1171	56 med
Goose, meat and skin roasted	301	1252	0 low
Graham crackers	465	1956	59 med
Grapefruit	30	126	25 low
Grapefruit juice, unsweetened	33	140	48 low
Grapes, red	60	257	53 low
Grapes, white	60	257	53 low
Green beans, raw	24	99	1 low
Green beans, steamed	25	108	1 low

H

	KCAL	KJ	GI VALUE
Haddock, steamed	89	378	0 low
Halibut, broiled	121	513	0 low
Ham	107	451	0 low

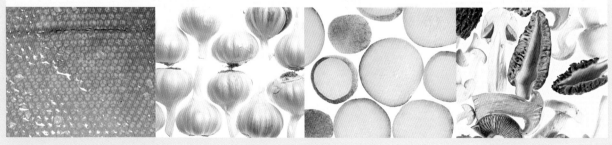

	KCAL	KJ	GI VALUE		KCAL	KJ	GI VALUE
Ham steak, fat removed, boiled	204	851	0 low	**Kidney beans,** soaked and boiled	100	424	28 low
Heart, lamb, roasted	226	944	0 low	**Kippers,** broiled	161	667	0 low
Herbal tea	0	0	0 low	**Kiwifruit**	49	207	53 low
Herbs, dried	181	760	1 low				
Herbs, fresh	34	141	1 low	**L**			
Honey	288	1229	55 low	**Lamb,** ground, stewed	208	870	0 low
Hummus	187	781	6 low	**Lamb,** kebab, broiled	288	1199	0 low
				Lamb, lean, roasted	203	853	0 low
I				**Lamb,** loin chop, lean broiled	213	892	0 low
Ice cream, full-fat	177	741	61 med	**Lamb,** loin chop, with fat broiled	277	1150	0 low
Ice cream, low-fat	119	499	50 low	**Lard**	891	3663	0 low
Instant mashed potato	57	245	86 high	**Leeks,** steamed	21	87	1 low
				Lentils, green canned	64	273	48 low
J				**Lentils,** green soaked and boiled	105	446	30 low
Jelly, apricot, reduced sugar	123	523	55 low	**Lentils,** red soaked and boiled	100	424	26 low
Jelly, strawberry	261	1114	56 med	**Lettuce,** iceberg	13	53	1 low
				Lettuce, round	14	59	1 low
K				**Lima beans,** canned	77	327	36 low
Kale, raw	33	140	1 low	**Lima beans,** soaked and cooked	103	437	31 low
Kale, steamed	24	100	1 low	**Liver, calf,** fried	188	784	0 low
Kidney, lamb, fried	188	784	0 low	**Liver, chicken,** fried	169	705	0 low
Kidney, ox, stewed	138	579	0 low	**Liver, lamb,** fried	237	989	0 low
Kidney, pig stewed and fried	153	641	0 low				
Kidney beans, canned	100	424	36 low				

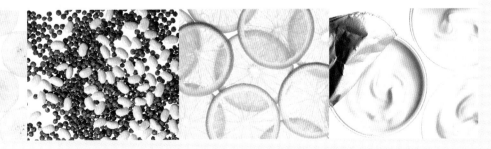

	KCAL	KJ	GI VALUE
Liver, ox, stewed	198	831	0 low
Liver pâté	348	1437	0 low
Lobster, boiled	103	435	0 low
Low-fat spread, 40% fat	390	1608	0 low
Low-fat spread, 75% fat	680	2795	0 low

M

	KCAL	KJ	GI VALUE
Mackerel, fresh, fried	272	1130	0 low
Mango	57	245	51 low
Margarine	718	2954	0 low
Mashed potato, instant	57	245	86 high
Meat extract	179	760	0 low

MEATS

	KCAL	KJ	GI VALUE
Bacon, broiled	337	1400	0 low
Bacon, Canadian broiled	287	1194	0 low
Bacon, Canadian reduced salt, broiled	282	1172	0 low
Beef, grillsteaks, broiled	305	1268	0 low
Beef, hamburgers, 99% meat, broiled	326	1353	0 low
Beef, round steak stewed	185	613	0 low
Beef, sirloin steak, lean fried	183	770	0 low
Beef, sirloin steak, lean grilled	177	745	0 low

	KCAL	KJ	GI VALUE
Beef, topround, lean and fat, roasted	222	930	0 low
Beef, corned, canned	205	860	0 low
Ham	107	451	0 low
Ham steak, fat removed, boiled	204	851	0 low
Kidney, lamb, fried	188	784	0 low
Kidney, ox, stewed	138	579	0 low
Kidney, pig, stewed and fried	153	641	0 low
Lamb, ground, stewed	208	870	0 low
Lamb, kebab, broiled	288	1199	0 low
Lamb, lean, roasted	203	853	0 low
Lamb, loin chop, lean broiled	213	892	0 low
Lamb, loin chop, with fat broiled	277	1150	0 low
Liver, calf, fried	188	784	0 low
Liver, chicken, fried	169	705	0 low
Liver, lamb, fried	237	989	0 low
Liver, ox, stewed	198	831	0 low
Liver pâté	348	1437	0 low
Pork, belly, grilled	320	1332	0 low
Pork, chop, lean and fat roasted	301	1256	0 low
Pork, leg, lean and fat roasted	182	765	0 low
Pork, loin chop, lean broiled	184	774	0 low

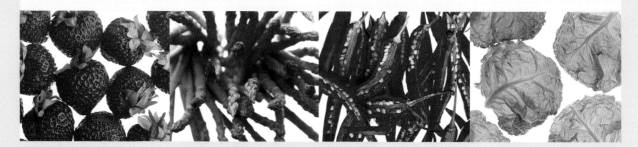

	KCAL	KJ	GI VALUE
Pork, steak, lean and fat broiled	198	832	0 low
Pork, tenderloin strips stir-fried	182	764	0 low
Sausages, pork, broiled	294	1221	28 low
Veal, scallop, fried	196	825	0 low
Veal, scallop, roasted	230	960	0 low
Venison, roasted	165	698	0 low

MILKS

	KCAL	KJ	GI VALUE
Condensed milk	333	1406	61 med
Skim milk	32	136	32 low
Soy milk	32	132	36 low
Soy yogurt	72	305	50 low
Whole milk	65	274	31 low
Mint, fresh	43	181	1 low
Mozzarella cheese	257	1067	0 low
Muesli, Swiss	363	1540	56 med
Multigrain bread	237	1005	61 med
Mushrooms, fried	157	645	1 low
Mushrooms, raw	13	55	1 low
Mussels, boiled, no shells	28	119	0 low
Mussels, boiled, with shells	104	440	0 low
Mustard, wholegrain	140	584	1 low
Mustard and cress	13	56	1 low

	KCAL	KJ	GI VALUE
N			
New potatoes, canned, reheated, and drained	66	281	65 med
New potatoes, unpeeled, boiled in their skins	75	321	76 high
O			
Oatcakes	412	1737	54 low

OILS AND FATS

	KCAL	KJ	GI VALUE
Butter	744	3059	0 low
Coconut oil	899	3696	0 low
Ghee	895	3693	0 low
Lard	891	3663	0 low
Low-fat spread, 40% fat	390	1608	0 low
Low-fat spread, 75% fat	680	2795	0 low
Margarine	718	2954	0 low
Olive oil	899	3696	0 low
Peanut/groundnut oil	899	3696	0 low
Sesame oil	899	3696	0 low
Sunflower oil	899	3696	0 low
Vegetable oil	899	3696	0 low
Okra, boiled	28	119	1 low
Okra, fried	269	1122	1 low
Olive oil	899	3696	0 low
Omelet, cheese	271	1121	0 low
Omelet, plain	195	808	0 low

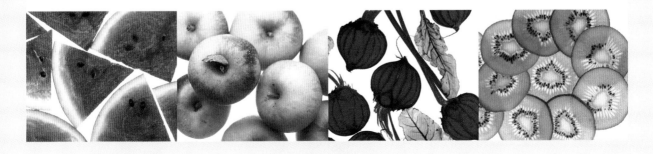

	KCAL	KJ	GI VALUE		KCAL	KJ	GI VALUE
Onions, fried	164	684	0 low	**Peaches,** canned in juice	39	165	40 low
Onions, raw	36	150	0 low	**Peanut/groundnut oil**	899	3696	0 low
Orange	37	158	42 low	**Peanuts,** dry roasted	589	2441	14 low
Orange juice, unsweetened	36	153	53 low	**Peanuts,** plain	563	2337	14 low
Oysters, raw	65	275	0 low	**Pears,** canned in juice	33	141	45 low
				Pecan nuts	689	2843	10 low

P

	KCAL	KJ	GI VALUE		KCAL	KJ	GI VALUE
Pancakes	302	1265	67 med	**Peeled potatoes,** boiled	72	306	101 high
Papaya	36	153	56 med	**Pepper,** black	0	0	0 low
Parmesan cheese	415	1729	0 low	**Pepper,** chili	20	83	1 low
Parsley, fresh	34	141	1 low	**Pepper,** white	0	0	0 low
				Peppers, bell, green, raw	15	65	1 low

PASTA, RICE AND GRAINS

	KCAL	KJ	GI VALUE		KCAL	KJ	GI VALUE
Barley, pearl, boiled	120	510	25 low	**Peppers, bell,** red, raw	32	134	1 low
Basmati rice, boiled	138	587	58 med	**Pheasant,** meat only roasted	220	918	0 low
Buckwheat, boiled	364	1522	54 low	**Pineapple,** canned in juice	47	200	46 low
Couscous, cooked	227	950	65 med	**Pineapple,** fresh	41	176	66 med
Egg noodles, boiled	62	264	46 low	**Pineapple juice,** unsweetened	41	177	46 low
Quinoa	309	1311	53 low	**Pita bread,** white	255	1084	57 med
Risotto rice, boiled	138	587	69 med	**Pizza,** cheese, thin-crust	277	1168	30 low
Spaghetti, brown, dried boiled	113	485	37 low	**Pizza,** cheese and tomato, deep-pan	249	1050	36 low
Spaghetti, white, boiled	104	442	38 low	**Pizza,** cheese and tomato, thin-crust	238	1003	36 low
White rice, boiled	138	587	98 high	**Pork belly,** grilled	320	1332	0 low
Pastry	451	1884	59 med	**Pork,** chop, lean and fat roasted	301	1256	0 low
Pâté, liver	348	1437	0 low				

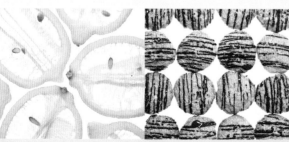
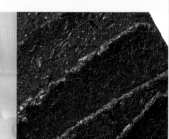

	KCAL	KJ	GI VALUE
Pork, leg, lean, roasted	182	765	0 low
Pork, loin chop, lean broiled	184	774	0 low
Pork, meat only, roasted	182	763	0 low
Pork, steak, lean and fat broiled	198	832	0 low
Pork, tenderloin strips, stir-fried	182	764	0 low

POTATOES

	KCAL	KJ	GI VALUE
Baked potato	136	581	85 high
Chips, potato	530	2215	57 med
Mashed potato, instant	57	245	86 high
New potatoes, canned, reheated, and drained	66	281	65 med
New potatoes, unpeeled, boiled in their skins	75	321	76 high
Peeled potatoes, boiled	72	306	101 high
Sweet potatoes, boiled	84	358	46 low

POULTRY AND GAME

	KCAL	KJ	GI VALUE
Chicken, breast, no skin broiled	148	626	0 low
Chicken, drumsticks roasted	185	775	0 low
Chicken, meat and skin roasted	216	912	0 low
Chicken, strips, stir-fried	161	677	0 low
Duck, crispy Chinese	331	1375	0 low

	KCAL	KJ	GI VALUE
Duck, meat and skin roasted	388	1603	0 low
Duck, meat only, roasted	195	815	0 low
Goose, meat and skin roasted	301	1252	0 low
Pheasant, meat only roasted	220	918	0 low
Rabbit, stewed	114	479	0 low
Turkey, breast, broiled	155	658	0 low
Turkey, meat and skin roasted	171	717	0 low
Turkey, strips, stir-fried	164	692	0 low

	KCAL	KJ	GI VALUE
Pretzels	381	1596	83 high
Prunes	141	601	29 low

Q

	KCAL	KJ	GI VALUE
Quinoa	309	1311	53 low
Quorn	86	360	1 low

R

	KCAL	KJ	GI VALUE
Rabbit, stewed	114	479	0 low
Radishes	12	49	1 low
Raisins	272	1159	64 med

RICE

	KCAL	KJ	GI VALUE
Basmati rice, boiled	138	587	58 med
Risotto rice, boiled	138	587	69 med
Rice cakes, white	374	1591	82 high

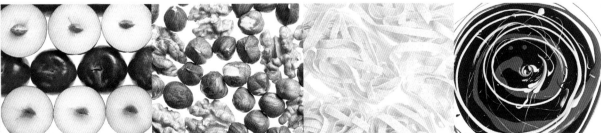

	KCAL	KJ	GI VALUE		KCAL	KJ	GI VALUE
Rice cereal, plain	382	1628	82 high				
Risotto rice, boiled	138	587	69 med				
Rolled oats, dried	401	1698	42 low				
Rye bread, no grains	219	932	51 low				
Rye/pumpernickel bread, with grains	219	932	41 low				

SNACKS (SAVORY)

	KCAL	KJ	GI VALUE
Chips, corn	459	1927	42 low
Chips, potato	530	2215	57 med
Peanuts, dry roasted	589	2441	14 low
Peanuts, plain	563	2337	14 low
Pretzels	381	1596	83 high
Rice cakes, white	374	1591	82 high

S

	KCAL	KJ	GI VALUE
Salami	438	1814	0 low
Salmon, canned in oil	153	644	0 low
Salmon, canned in brine	153	644	0 low
Salmon, fresh, steamed	194	812	0 low
Salmon, smoked	142	598	0 low
Salt	0	0	0 low
Sardines, canned in oil	220	918	0 low
Sardines, fresh, broiled	195	815	0 low
Sausages, pork, broiled	294	1221	28 low
Scallops, steamed	118	501	0 low
Scones, plain	364	1530	92 high
Sesame oil	899	3696	0 low
Shortbread	509	2133	64 med
Shrimp, canned in brine	94	398	0 low
Shrimp, frozen	73	310	0 low
Shrimp, peeled and boiled	99	418	0 low
Skim milk	32	136	32 low

SNACKS (SWEET)

	KCAL	KJ	GI VALUE
Chocolate, dark	510	2137	41 low
Chocolate, milk	520	2177	49 low
Chocolate mousse	149	627	37 low
Chocolate mousse, low-fat	123	518	31 low
Graham crackers	465	1956	59 med
Ice cream, full-fat	177	741	61 med
Ice cream, low-fat	119	499	50 low
Shortbread	509	2133	64 med
Sponge cake	467	1951	46 low
Yogurt, low-fat	56	237	33 low
Yogurt, low-fat, fruit	78	331	31 low
Yogurt, virtually fat-free, diet	54	230	20 low

	KCAL	KJ	GI VALUE
Snow peas, raw	32	136	1 low
Snow peas, steamed	26	111	1 low
Snow peas, stir-fried	71	298	1 low
Sole fillet, steamed	91	384	0 low

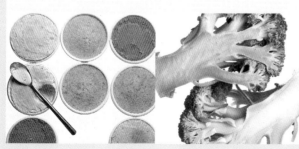

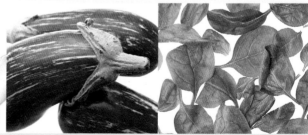

	KCAL	KJ	GI VALUE		KCAL	KJ	GI VALUE
Soy beans, cooked	141	590	20 low				
Soy/linseed bread	252	1070	41 low	**T**			
Soy milk	32	132	36 low	**Tea,** black	0	0	0 low
Soy sauce	43	182	1 low	**Tempeh**	166	697	10 low
Soy yogurt	72	305	50 low	**Tofu,** fried	261	1086	1 low
Spaghetti, brown, dried boiled	113	485	37 low	**Tofu,** steamed	73	304	1 low
Spaghetti, white, boiled	104	442	38 low	**Tomato juice,** no added sugar	14	62	38 low
Spinach, raw	25	103	1 low	**Tomato soup,** canned	52	219	45 low
Spinach, steamed	19	79	1 low	**Trout fillet,** broiled	135	565	0 low
Split peas, soaked and cooked	126	538	32 low	**Tuna,** canned in brine	99	422	0 low
Sponge cake	467	1951	46 low	**Tuna,** canned in oil	189	794	0 low
				Tuna pâté	236	986	0 low
SPREADS AND DIPS				**Turkey,** breast, broiled	155	658	0 low
Honey	288	1229	55 low	**Turkey,** meat and skin roasted	171	717	0 low
Hummus	187	781	6 low	**Turkey,** strips, stir-fried	164	692	0 low
Jelly, apricot, reduced sugar	123	523	55 low				
Jelly, strawberry	261	1114	56 med	**V**			
				Veal, scallop, fried	196	825	0 low
Stilton cheese	410	1698	0 low	**Veal,** scallop, roasted	230	960	0 low
Stuffing, sage and onion	269	1126	74 high	**Vegetable oil**	899	3696	0 low
Sugar	394	1680	68 med				
Sunflower oil	899	3696	0 low	**VEGETABLES**			
Sweet potatoes, boiled	87	372	44 low	**Artichoke,** boiled	18	77	1 low
Swordfish, broiled	139	583	0 low	**Artichoke,** canned	28	119	1 low
				Asparagus, steamed	26	110	1 low
				Avocado	190	784	1 low

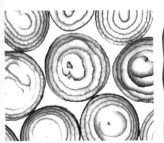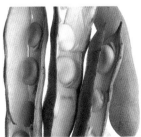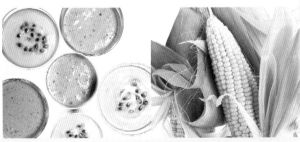

	KCAL	KJ	GI VALUE		KCAL	KJ	GI VALUE
Bean sprouts, raw	31	131	1 low	**Leeks,** steamed	21	87	1 low
Bean sprouts, stir-fried	72	298	1 low	**Lettuce,** round	14	59	1 low
				Lettuce, iceberg	13	53	1 low
Beet, boiled	36	154	64 med	**Mushrooms,** fried	157	645	1 low
Broccoli, green, raw	33	138	1 low	**Mushrooms,** raw	13	55	1 low
Broccoli, green, steamed	24	100	1 low	**Mustard and cress**	13	56	1 low
Brussels sprouts, steamed	35	153	1 low	**Okra,** boiled	28	119	1 low
Cabbage, raw	26	109	1 low	**Okra,** fried	269	1122	1 low
Cabbage, steamed	16	67	1 low	**Onions,** fried	164	684	0 low
Carrots, raw	35	146	49 low	**Onions,** raw	36	150	0 low
Carrots, steamed	24	100	31 low	**Pepper,** chili	20	83	1 low
Cauliflower, boiled	28	117	1 low	**Peppers, bell,** green, raw	15	65	1 low
Cauliflower, raw	34	142	1 low	**Peppers, bell,** red, raw	32	134	1 low
Celery, raw	7	30	0 low	**Radishes**	12	49	1 low
Celery, steamed	8	34	0 low	**Snow peas,** raw	32	136	1 low
Collard greens, raw	33	136	1 low	**Snow peas,** steamed	26	111	1 low
Collard greens, steamed	20	82	1 low	**Snow peas,** stir-fried	71	298	1 low
Corn, boiled	66	280	48 low	**Spinach,** raw	25	103	1 low
Corn, canned	23	96	46 low	**Spinach,** steamed	19	79	1 low
Cucumber	10	40	1 low	**Sweet potatoes,** boiled	84	358	46 low
Eggplant, fried	302	1246	1 low	**Tomato juice,** no added sugar	14	62	38 low
Fennel, boiled	11	47	1 low				
Fennel, raw	12	50	1 low	**Watercress**	22	94	1 low
Green beans, raw	24	99	1 low	**Yam,** boiled	133	568	37 low
Green beans, steamed	25	108	1 low	**Zucchini,** fried	62	265	1 low
Kale, raw	33	140	1 low	**Zucchini,** raw	18	74	1 low
Kale, steamed	24	100	1 low	**Zucchini,** steamed	19	81	1 low

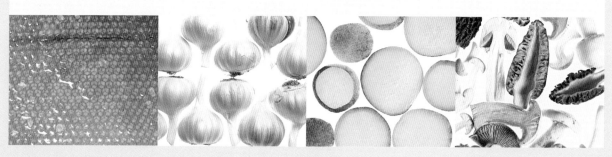

	KCAL	KJ	GI VALUE		KCAL	KJ	GI VALUE
Veggieburger, broiled	196	821	59 med	**Y**			
Venison, roasted	165	698	0 low	**Yam,** boiled	133	568	37 low
Vinegar	22	89	0 low	**Yeast extract**	180	763	0 low
				Yogurt, low-fat	56	237	33 low
W				**Yogurt,** low-fat, fruit	78	331	31 low
Waffles	334	1401	76 high	**Yogurt,** virtually fat-free, diet	54	230	20 low
Water	0	0	0 low				
Water biscuits	440	1859	77 high	**Z**			
Watercress	22	94	1 low	**Zucchini,** fried	62	265	1 low
Watermelon, no skin	31	133	72 high	**Zucchini,** raw	18	74	1 low
Weetabix	352	1498	69 med	**Zucchini,** steamed	19	81	1 low
Wheat cereal	89	376	0 low				
White bread	235	1002	70 high				
White rice, cooked	138	587	98 high				
Whiting, steamed	92	406	0 low				
Whole milk	66	274	31 low				
Whole-wheat bread	217	922	77 high				
Worcestershire sauce	65	276	1 low				

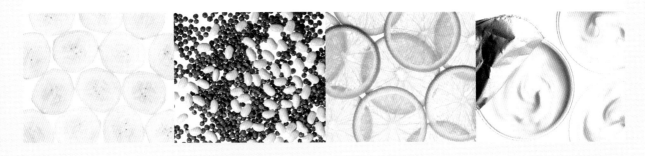

Index

Executive editor: Nicola Hill
Project editor: Alice Bowden
Deputy creative director: Geoff Fennell
Designer: Ginny Zeal

Photography: Will Heap, Mike Prior, Ian O'Leary, Gareth Sambidge
Home economist: Sara Lewis
Senior production controller: Martin Croshaw